Walking Baltimore

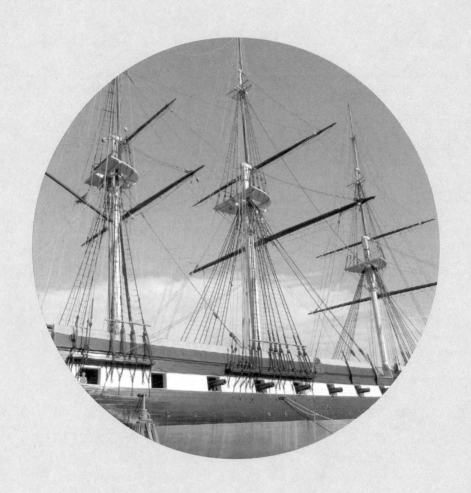

WALKING BALTIMORE

An Insider's Guide to 33 Historic Neighborhoods, Waterfront Districts, and Hidden Treasures in Charm City

Evan Balkan

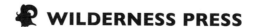 WILDERNESS PRESS

Walking Baltimore: An Insider's Guide to 33 Historic Neighborhoods, Waterfront Districts, and Hidden Treasures in Charm City

1st EDITION 2013

Copyright © 2013 by Evan Balkan

Cover and interior photos by Evan Balkan
Maps: Scott McGrew
Cover and book design: Larry B. Van Dyke and Lisa Pletka
Book layout: Annie Long
Book editor: Holly Cross

ISBN 978-0-89997-701-0

Manufactured in the United States of America

Published by: **Wilderness Press**
Keen Communications
PO Box 43673
Birmingham, AL 35243
(800) 443-7227; FAX (205) 326-1012
info@wildernesspress.com
www.wildernesspress.com

Visit our website for a complete listing of our books and for ordering information.

Distributed by Publishers Group West

Cover photos: Front, clockwise from upper right: Sherwood Gardens, Guilford; Washington Monument, Mount Vernon Place; Painted Ladies, Charles Village; Mr. Boh, Brewers Hill; National Aquarium, Inner Harbor; Orianda House, Leakin Park; Orpheus statue, Fort McHenry. *Back, top to bottom:* Francis Scott Key Monument, Bolton Hill; Moorish Tower, Druid Hill Park; Maryland Institute College of Art, Mount Royal.

Frontispiece: USS *Constellation*; see Walk 4: Inner Harbor Promenade, page 23

SAFETY NOTICE: Although Wilderness Press and the author have made every attempt to ensure that the information in this book is accurate at press time, they are not responsible for any loss, damage, injury, or inconvenience that may occur to anyone while using this book. You are responsible for your own safety and health while following the walking trips described here. Always check local conditions, know your own limitations, and consult a map.

author's note

I was not born in Baltimore and so don't have any innate hometown bias. In fact, having grown up in Washington, D.C., and coming from a family of New Yorkers, I used to regard Baltimore with distant reproach (until I actually got to know the place and decided to make my home here). I've been fortunate to have traveled in some 25 foreign countries and at least as many states; my regard for Charm City does not come from not knowing anything different. To my continued surprise, I've come to see Baltimore as one of the great cities anywhere. It's not surprising then that this book has been a joy to write; it has served as a constant reminder of why I love this city so much. This is a place where people are primarily interested in honesty and authenticity. Here, you are free to be what you will be.

Baltimore, for all its worldly attributes and 3 million metro residents, can often feel like a provincial place, what some derisively call Smalltimore. Baltimore is a patchwork of small, unique neighborhoods. But there's something simply nice about that, isn't there? This is a city where you can feel part of a real place (no pretense in Baltimore—no way), a community, where you are bound to bump into someone you know. And as it happens, in perhaps the country's largest small town, you will find all the amenities that make Baltimore a world-class city, a place that can often feel much bigger than it is. It's this dichotomy that makes Baltimore endlessly interesting, a place of constant reinvention. But some things invariably stay the same: the neighborhoods and the people who make up those neighborhoods.

Whether you know the city well or are a first-time visitor, use this book as a guide through these unique neighborhoods. You'll be amazed at how much is here. And use your feet. Walking the streets, in the paths of history and culture, you'll soon see why Baltimore easily lives up to its nickname, Charm City.

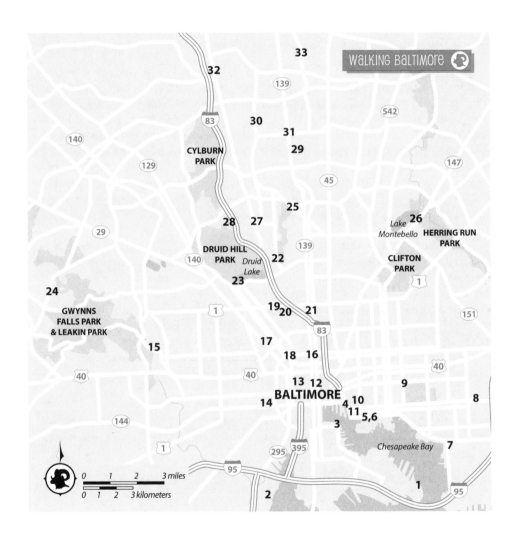

WALKING BALTIMORE

33

32

139

83

30

31

29

139

542

CYLBURN PARK

140

129

147

45

25

29

28 27

Lake Montebello 26 HERRING RUN PARK

DRUID HILL PARK

140

22

139

Druid Lake

CLIFTON PARK

24

23

1

GWYNNS FALLS PARK & LEAKIN PARK

1

19 20 21

151

83

15

17

18 16

40

40

40

13 12

9

8

BALTIMORE

14

4 10

11 5,6

3

144

Chesapeake Bay

7

1

1

395

295

1

83

2

95

95

0 1 2 3 miles

0 1 2 3 kilometers

NUMBERS ON THIS LOCATOR MAP CORRESPOND TO WALK NUMBERS.

TaBLe OF CONTENTS

INTRODUCTION

Ask people around the country what they think of when they think of Baltimore and you might hear something about baseball or Johns Hopkins or something else positive, but there's a decent chance that what you'll hear won't be so great. The national image of Baltimore has taken a hit, thanks to popular shows like *The Wire,* a show focusing on Baltimore's drug underworld. Yes, there are problems here; *The Wire* isn't pure fiction. But those who know this city intimately know there is so much more (after all, the creator of *The Wire* still chooses to live here). In fact, this duality is one of the things that makes Baltimore such a distinctive place. So often it has been the case that when playing unofficial tour guide to out-of-town visitors, I hear them frequently remark with admiration, "I had no idea," when I point out some piece of history or take them to a great neighborhood far off the beaten path. This is a city that constantly surprises and a city that has it all: terrific cultural institutions, wonderful bars and restaurants, and more recreation and green space than most people realize. There is a reason the colonial settlers built a town here: Baltimore enjoys a special geographic spot, sandwiched between the Alleghenies to the west and the Atlantic Ocean to the east and sitting atop the country's largest estuary. It enjoys four seasons, moderate temperature, and quick and easy access to all the things that make living in the Mid-Atlantic such a pleasure. It's not for nothing that Baltimore and its environs have been called The Land of Pleasant Living. So let others cling to a one-sided or negative view. Let them reduce this great city to what they see on TV. We lucky ones can see all the things that make Baltimore one of the world's great places.

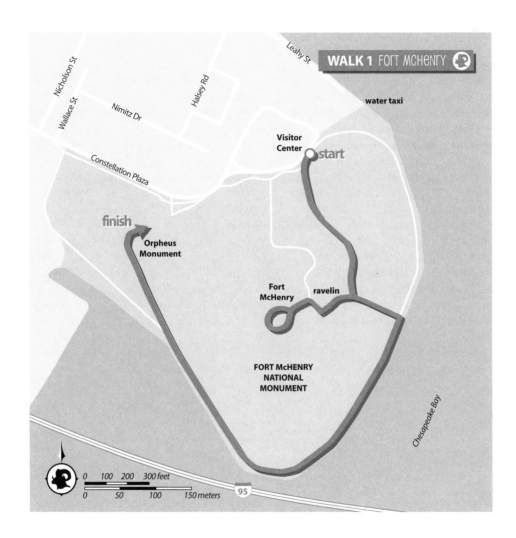

Leahy St

Nicholson St

Wallace St

Nimitz Dr

Halsey Rd

water taxi

Visitor
Center

start

Constellation Plaza

finish

Orpheus
Monument

Fort
McHenry

ravelin

FORT McHENRY
NATIONAL
MONUMENT

Chesapeake Bay

0   100   200   300 feet

0   50   100   150 meters

95

1 FORT MCHENRY: STAR-SPANGLED GLORY

BOUNDARIES: **Constellation Plaza, sea wall**
DISTANCE: **> 1 mile**
DIFFICULTY: **Easy**
PARKING: **In the lot at Constellation Plaza, in front of the visitor center**
PUBLIC TRANSIT: **MTA bus #1, Water Taxi #17**

This is a short walk that's long on history and rather unforgettable as a result. It was here that Francis Scott Key, one of Maryland's most famous native sons, penned the poem that would become the American national anthem. Fearing a British attack after our Declaration of Independence, the citizens of Baltimore hastily constructed an earthen fort, Fort Whetstone, on the banks of the Patapsco River. The attack never materialized, but the spot continued to be recognized as particularly strategic. Construction on a more permanent fort with masonry walls began in 1798 and was completed in 1803. It was named after James McHenry, America's second Secretary of War. It was in the War of 1812 that the fort shined brightest and gave Americans a rallying point that stirs emotions to this day. The feared British attack from decades earlier materialized on September 13–14, 1814. The British had already marched on Washington, burned the Capitol, and now set their sights on Baltimore, then America's third-largest city and occupying a prime location. Key, on a British warship in the harbor to negotiate the release of Marylander Dr. William Beanes, listened to the bombardment through the night and was shocked and thrilled to see the American flag, that "star-spangled banner," still waving come morning. One thousand brave Americans had repelled the attack, and the fledging nation was on its way to a future of unprecedented prosperity and might. Today Fort McHenry is the only attraction in the National Park System administered as both a Historic Shrine and a National Monument.

● **Begin in the gleaming new $15 million visitor center, constructed in 2011, in time for the 200th anniversary of the Battle of Baltimore. The original visitor center was built in 1964 and was designed to accommodate some 150,000 tourists. But the site eventually came to regularly attract upwards of 650,000 visitors per year. Now, with the wonderful new structure and the bicentennial of the battle approaching, the National Park Service expects that Fort McHenry could soon start seeing a million or more visitors a year.**

Back Story

Despite its being the national anthem of the United States, the lyrics to "The Star-Spangled Banner" are unknown to most Americans beyond the first verse. Here, then, is the poem as Key penned it:

O say can you see . . . by the dawn's early light,
What so proudly we hail'd at the twilight's last gleaming
Whose broad stripes and bright stars, through the perilous fight,
O'er the ramparts we watch'd, were so gallantly streaming?
And the rocket's red glare, the bombs bursting in air,
Gave proof through the night that our flag was still there,
O say does that star-spangled banner yet wave
O'er the land of the free and the home of the brave?

On the shore dimly seen through the mists of the deep
Where the foe's haughty host in dread silence reposes,
What is that which the breeze, o'er the towering steep,
As it fitfully blows, half conceals, half discloses?
Now it catches the gleam of the morning's first beam,
In full glory reflected now shines in the stream,
'Tis the star-spangled banner—O long may it wave
O'er the land of the free and the home of the brave!

And where is that band who so vauntingly swore
That the havoc of war and the battle's confusion
A home and a Country should leave us no more?
Their blood has wash'd out their foul footsteps' pollution.
No refuge could save the hireling and slave
From the terror of flight or the gloom of the grave,
And the star-spangled banner in triumph doth wave
O'er the land of the free and the home of the brave.

O thus be it ever when freemen shall stand
Between their lov'd home and the war's desolation!
Blest with vict'ry and peace may the heav'n-rescued land
Praise the power that hath made and preserv'd us a nation!
Then conquer we must, when our cause it is just,
And this be our motto—"In God is our trust,"
And the star-spangled banner in triumph shall wave
O'er the land of the free and the home of the brave.

The new center is a beauty. A two-story LEED-certified (Leadership in Energy and Environmental Design) building, it houses artifacts, a bronze statue of Francis Scott Key (conspicuously missing from the previous visitor center), and a wonderful film with an ending that could stir even the most hardened heart. The original manuscript of Key's famous poem was on loan for the first few months after the visitor center's grand opening, but to see it now, you'll have to visit the Maryland Historical Society. That's easy enough to do; just follow Walk 16: Mt. Vernon.

- When you're through at the visitor center, walk onto the grounds. Follow the path from the back of the visitor center toward the V-shaped wedge sitting opposite the fort. This is the ravelin, designed to protect the fort's entrance from direct attack.

- Opposite the ravelin in the arched entryway, you'll notice underground rooms to either side of the entrance. These originally served as bombproofs but doubled as powder magazines during the Civil War.

- Just ahead are the parade grounds and flagpole. Flag-changing ceremonies take place each day at 9:30 a.m. and 4:20 p.m. Tradition holds that each new official American flag (to commemorate the inclusion into the Union of Alaska or Hawaii, for example) is flown first at Fort McHenry, before anywhere else in the country.

The fort as you see it today doesn't look exactly as it did when it was built more than 200 years ago. The years have seen many additions and improvements to suit evolving needs; indeed, the fort has served changing national interests from the start. After its prominent role in the War of 1812, Fort McHenry became home to training soldiers for the war with Mexico in 1846–1848. Fifteen years later, Confederate soldiers were housed at Fort McHenry during the Civil War; the numbers were usually in the lower hundreds but swelled to nearly 7,000 after the Battle of Gettysburg. In 1912, 100 years after its greatest glory, Fort McHenry closed as a military training center. The 141st Coastal Artillery Company had the distinction of being the last military unit garrisoned at the fort. But Fort McHenry saw renewed action as a military hospital for returning WWI soldiers, as U.S. Army Hospital No. 2, at the time the largest receiving hospital in the country, employing almost a thousand medical professionals. Fort McHenry saw a major restoration in the 1930s by the Works Progress Administration. The restoration work that this New Deal program accomplished is what one sees at the fort today. The National Park Service took over operations of Fort McHenry in 1933. But even then, Fort McHenry's service to America wasn't complete. The U.S. Coast Guard used the fort for port security during WWII.

● Working your way from left to right from the flagpole, you will see five separate buildings. The first two buildings are soldiers' barracks, housing the 60-man garrisons stationed there. Next up is the junior officers' quarters. The building with the semicircular roof is the powder magazine. During the battle, a massive British bomb struck the magazine, but fortunately the bomb did not explode, which spared hundreds of lives. Last up is the commanding officer's quarters, which was used by Major George Armistead, still a Baltimore legend. He's buried in Old St. Paul's Cemetery in Baltimore. It was Armistead who ordered the installation at the fort of the massive American flag (42 by 30 feet; each stripe was 2 feet wide, and the stars measured 2 feet each from point to point). Today's replica is just as large and carries the 15 stars and 15 stripes of the day, one for each state in the Union at the time. Look for Armistead's bronze monument near the visitor center. Another Armistead monument stands atop Federal Hill (see Walk 3). Each building contains artifacts and historical notes.

● Continue on the trail outside of the fort toward the seawall. Once you reach the edge of the Patapsco River, you can go left if you wish to make a complete circuit and take the shortest route back to the visitor center. However, I'd recommend heading right, which will give you a longer walk and take you to the massive Orpheus statue.

● As you walk along the sea wall, take time to enjoy the view: the Patapsco spreading into the Chesapeake Bay; the Key Bridge off in the distance; the industry of south Baltimore. If it's summer, the inevitable breeze coming off the water will offer instant refreshment. But beware: in winter, this breeze can bite.

● There will be no mistaking it when you reach the Orpheus monument; it's enormous. Though Orpheus was the Greek god of music and poetry, this monument is actually to Francis Scott Key. You'll notice depictions of Key around the base of the statue. It was on the occasion of the dedication of this monument in 1922 that Warren Harding became the first president to be broadcast on radio coast to coast.

POINT OF INTEREST (START TO FINISH)

Fort McHenry National Monument and Historic Shrine
nps.gov/fomc, 2400 E. Fort Ave., 410-962-4290

ROUTE SUMMARY

1. Begin at the Fort McHenry Visitor Center.
2. Tour the fort and grounds.
3. Circle the sea wall.

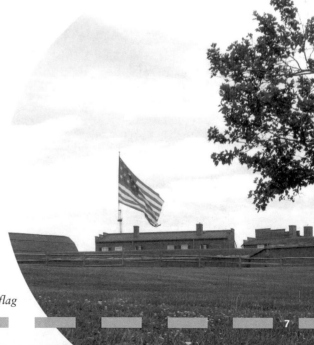

Fort McHenry and massive American flag

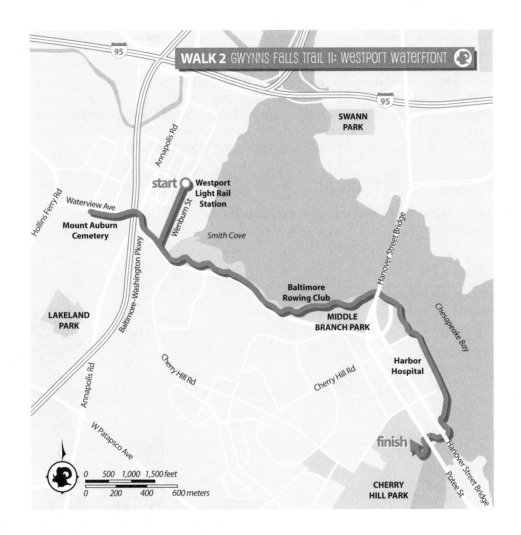

SWANN
PARK

Annapolis Rd

I-95

I-95

Hollins Ferry Rd

Waterview Ave

start ⭕ Westport
Light Rail
Station

Wenburn St

Smith Cove

Mount Auburn
Cemetery

Baltimore-Washington Pkwy

LAKELAND
PARK

Baltimore
Rowing Club

MIDDLE
BRANCH PARK

Hanover Street Bridge

Chesapeake Bay

Harbor
Hospital

Cherry Hill Rd

Cherry Hill Rd

Annapolis Rd

W Patapsco Ave

0   500   1,000 1,500 feet
0   200   400   600 meters

finish

Hanover Street Bridge

Potee St.

CHERRY
HILL PARK

2 GWYNNS FaLLS TraiL II: WesTPorT WaTerFronT

BOUNDARIES: Wenburn St./Kloman St., Gwynns Falls Trail, Potee St./Cherry Hill Park
DISTANCE: 1.8 miles one way
DIFFICULTY: Easy to moderate
PARKING: Harbor Hospital (see below), Wenburn St.
PUBLIC TRANSIT: Westport Light Rail, Cherry Hill Light Rail, and MTA buses #27 and #29 run east–west along Waterview Ave. MTA buses #27 and #64 run north–south on S. Hanover St.

Westport and neighboring Cherry Hill often stick in the minds of many Baltimoreans as marginal neighborhoods, teetering on an abyss. Indeed, a stroll through the residential sections of these neighborhoods reveals a lot of abandoned houses. However, a $1.5-billion development package is in the works for waterfront Westport that promises to change the very face of this area in a major way. The aim is to capitalize on Westport's location next to I-95 (easy access to D.C. and Maryland's central corridor) and its proximity to downtown. If the plans are realized, Westport could soon be the sort of place that every Baltimorean knows in a way very different from now. We can hope that all the coming change and prosperity will spill over into Cherry Hill as well. This walk begins at the site of the coming caravanserai and traverses the Gwynns Falls Trail along the Patapsco River, taking in the views and the attributes that make the area so ripe for revitalization.

Note: For a thorough description/explanation of the Gwynns Falls Trail, see Walk 15: Gwynns Falls Trail: From Leon Day to Mount Clare.

● Begin at the Westport Light Rail station. When you get off, the Middle Branch of the Patapsco River will be right in front of you to the east. Behind you, just a bit to the south, is the intersection of Cedley St. and Kent. St. You can head into the residential section of Westport just a block to 2222 Cedley St. to see where Al Kaline, Detroit Tigers slugger and baseball Hall of Famer, was born. Kaline's father worked at a nearby broom factory, while his mother scrubbed the factory floors. The Tigers drafted him in 1954, signing him for $35,000, a record amount for baseball in those days.

● Between the water and the Light Rail station is Wenburn St. Take it heading south (right if you're facing the water; Wenburn heading north becomes Kloman St.). At the time of this writing, the area parallel to Wenburn St. is a massive open area of cranes and bulldozers. What's coming here is something truly extraordinary. But first, what used to be here:

The area's industrial beginning dates to 1773, when John Moale built an iron furnace at the mouth of the Gwynns Falls where it spills into the Patapsco. Many of the foundry workers were African American, both freedmen and slaves. By the 1800s, Westport was growing, with several major rail lines—B&O, Western Maryland, Annapolis Short Line—running through the neighborhood. In the 19th century, this area was popular for city dwellers to swim, fish, crab, and boat. Shad, herring, perch, rockfish, and soft-shell crabs were abundant. In 1889, Carr & Lowrey set up a glass factory on the 16-acre parcel just north of where you stand now; mostly second-generation German immigrants filled those jobs. Soon after, Baltimore Gas & Electric's predecessor, Consolidated Gas, Electric Light & Power, built the massive Westport Power Station; at the time it was the largest reinforced-concrete power-generating station in the world, also a bit north of where you are now. All this industry required workers, and the housing stock to accommodate soon followed. The residential neighborhood of Westport, behind you, was built primarily in the 1920s. Jobs were abundant, and residents of Westport enjoyed shops and services after Baltimore City annexed the neighborhood. Westport, for better or worse, had a distinctive identity compared to neighboring Cherry Hill to the south: Westport for whites, Cherry Hill for blacks. But as the 20th century wore on, many of the industrial jobs began to disappear. Today's I-295, the Baltimore–Washington Parkway, built in the 1950s, split Westport in half. Soon after, white residents left for the suburbs, and Westport, like Cherry Hill, became overwhelmingly black (more than 90% of the population today) and increasingly poor and neglected. Some 20% of the housing in the neighborhood was vacant as of 2010. But because the neighborhood sits so near water, and because that shoreline is five times the size of the Inner Harbor, Baltimore's jewel, its redevelopment seems as obvious as it is essential. The city has partnered with private developers, and both parties have invested great sums of money into transforming Westport. There are still many families in Westport who care a great deal for their neighborhood and desperately want improvements.

● Look northeast, over the water, and you will see the swing bridge across the Middle Branch. It was used for CSX rail. The novel, swinging structure allowed ships to pass

without requiring a drawbridge. The plans for the CSX swing bridge include incorpo-
ration as a 5-mile hike-and-bike trail, to link with the Gwynns Falls Trail (GFT). North
of the bridge, a planned 236-foot sculpture will be, if realized, the largest contemporary sculpture on the continent, dramatically altering Baltimore's skyline. The sculptor,
John Henry, developed a fondness for Baltimore after undergoing surgery at Johns
Hopkins Hospital. Between the bridge and Waterview Ave., to the south—where you're
headed next—will be the extraordinary Westport Waterfront.

The development plan involves 50 acres and $1.5 billion. The goal is to have the
entire neighborhood LEED (Leadership in Energy and Environmental Design) plati-
num certified for Neighborhood Development, a first on the East Coast. The LEED
designation depends upon many factors, such as housing density, wetlands conser-
vation, public transportation, and energy efficiency—all areas where Westport excels.
Light Rail is already in place, of course, and easy access to waterfront also plays a
large part in the plans. Middle Branch Park and the GFT are integral to city plans for
the entire Middle Branch region to serve as a future green and environmentally conscious gateway to south Baltimore. A planned 8-acre forest-conservation area with
some 70,000 new trees will aid in this effort. As for the development itself, there will
be some 2,000 apartments, condos, and town homes, plus 3 million square feet of
office space, 300,000 square feet of retail, and 500 hotel rooms.

Part of the plan is to have the developer also work on existing housing stock in
Westport. In other words, what the city and other interested parties are trying to
avoid is to have a brand new gleaming playground for wealthy folks while leaving
the blight in Westport alone. Already, there have been substantial improvements
along Westport's main street, Annapolis Road. Also, a significant percentage of the
new development will be classified as affordable so that some existing residents of
Westport and neighboring Cherry Hill can live in the new housing.

●   Take a right on Wenburn St. and follow it to a left onto Waterview Ave. The GFT parallels Waterview Ave. Just 500 feet to the west is historic Mount Auburn Cemetery;
it's not a terribly pleasant walk there, but it might be worth checking out. Recently
cleared and finally cared for after many years of neglect, Mount Auburn was once
known as the City of the Dead for Colored People. It contains 55,000 graves of
African Americans and dates to 1872, when cemeteries were segregated, making

it one of the oldest "colored" graveyards in the country. Many prominent African Americans are buried there.

- At Cherry Hill Rd., the trail splits away from Waterview Ave. and heads toward the water. The change from urban to wetland is as dramatic as it is swift as you here enter 27-acre Middle Branch Park. John Smith, founder of the Jamestown colony, passed through here in 1608. Take the wooden wildlife observation boardwalk from the GFT to the viewing deck over Smith Cove. The area is lovely and green, surrounded by milkweed, cattails, goldenrod, and wildflowers. There are always many water birds about as well—a somewhat incongruous but pleasing sight against the backdrop of the city skyline. The Middle Branch acts as a migratory stop on the Atlantic Flyway, so keep your eyes open for non-native avian visitors. As noted, there will be further buffering of wetlands, plus the installation of two new piers specially designed as put-ins for kayakers and crew. There's another observation deck to the right.

- Head back to the GFT and go left, following the trail as it emerges from the trees and parallels the Middle Branch, soon coming to the Middle Branch Marina. Just beyond, in the red-roofed building, is the home of the Baltimore Rowing Club (baltimorerowing .org). Follow the path as it winds along the water, passing picnic benches and shade trees. Across the water from the marina is the proposed spot for a $50 million expansion of the National Aquarium in Baltimore. The 20-acre site will include an aquatic-life center, a park, and a fishing pier. Animal-care operations, classrooms, and research space will also be part of the future development.

- Continuing along the GFT through Middle Branch Park, you'll soon come to the distinctive Hanover Street Bridge (renamed the Vietnam Veterans Memorial Bridge in 1993). This 1916 Beaux Arts drawbridge connects Port Covington/Locust Point and Cherry Hill, the north and south banks of the Middle Branch. Apart from its utility as an important city roadway, the bridge has four attractive towers, one on each corner. The hike-and-bike trail that will take in the CSX swing bridge will incorporate Hanover Street Bridge to create a 5-mile loop.

- Go under the Hanover Street Bridge as the GFT cuts through Broening Park and passes the Broening Boat Ramp just beyond, yielding to a lovely little section that continues to wind along the edge of the Patapsco. Broening Park used to be home to the Baltimore Yacht Club, which held competitive races in these waters, events many Baltimoreans attended. To the right is Harbor Hospital, buffered by a hill of wildflowers. *Note:* There's parking available at Harbor Hospital, so you can arrive by car and do this walk in reverse. To do so, take I-95 to Exit 54, Hanover St. Go over the Hanover Street Bridge and turn left at Cherry Hill Rd. or Reedbird Ave. The parking lot is at 3001 S. Hanover St.

There's a bit more of the GFT left in this area. (Future plans call for linking it with trails that head into Annapolis, such as the B&A Trail, as well as linking it with Masonville Cove in Brooklyn to the south. All of this is part of the East Coast Greenway, a network of trails running from Maine to Florida.) You'll notice a few more fishing piers near S. Hanover St. as the GFT moves under the bridge and under Potee St., and then emerges into Cherry Hill Park. Across the water is Reed Bird Island Park. Here is where you'll need to turn around and retrace your steps to your starting point.

POINTS OF INTEREST (START TO FINISH)

Westport Waterfront westportwaterfront.com, 410-685-0250

Gwynns Falls Trail gwynnsfallstrail.org, 410-448-5663, ext. 135

Middle Branch Park middlebranchbaltimore .com

Hanover Street/Vietnam Veterans Memorial Bridge Hanover St.

ROUTE SUMMARY

1. Start at the Westport Light Rail station.
2. Turn right onto Wenburn St.
3. Turn left onto Waterview Ave.
4. Pick up the Gwynns Falls Trail.
5. Follow the Gwynns Falls Trail to Cherry Hill Park.

Patapsco River from Middle Branch Park

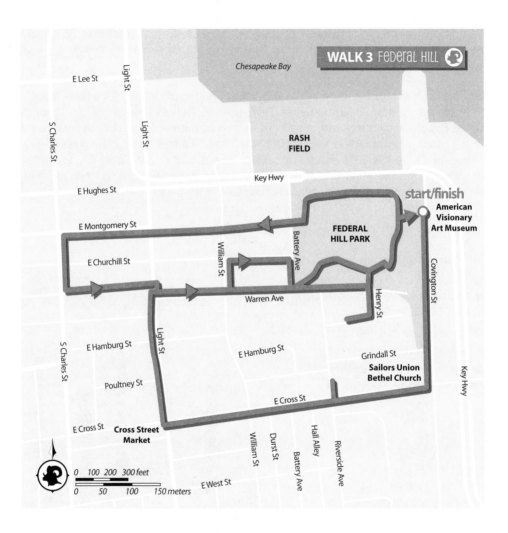

Chesapeake Bay

E Lee St

Light St

S Charles St

Light St

RASH FIELD

E Hughes St

Key Hwy

E Montgomery St

start/finish

American Visionary Art Museum

FEDERAL HILL PARK

Battery Ave

Covington St

E Churchill St

William St

Warren Ave

Henry St

Light St

E Hamburg St

E Hamburg St

Grindall St

Sailors Union Bethel Church

Key Hwy

Poultney St

E Cross St

E Cross St

Cross Street Market

William St

Durst St

Battery Ave

Hall Alley

Riverside Ave

E West St

0   100 200 300 feet

0   50   100   150 meters

3 Federal Hill: South Baltimore's 400-Year-Old Anchor

BOUNDARIES: **Covington St./Key Hwy., Cross St., S. Charles St., E. Montgomery St.**
DISTANCE: **1.9 miles**
DIFFICULTY: **Moderate**
PARKING: **Street parking with residential restrictions and limitations along route**
PUBLIC TRANSIT: **MTA bus #64 runs along Light St.**

Federal Hill encompasses some of South Baltimore's oldest architecture. This part of the city has hosted folks since well back in the 18th century, having first been sighted by John Smith more than 400 years ago. The street names in Federal Hill all seem to carry a whiff of Revolutionary War times. When mining, canning, and manufacturing moved in, these industries left Federal Hill a somewhat rundown neighborhood that nevertheless managed to ooze character and a certain blue-collar grace. For many locals, it was here, on the hills above the harbor, that the "real Baltimore" clung tenaciously for decades. Today, Federal Hill is a trendy destination, with some of those rehabbed 18th- and 19th-century houses on cobblestone streets fetching small fortunes. With the addition of a plethora of shops and restaurants, plus one of the coolest museums anywhere—and, of course, the best views in the city—Federal Hill seems poised to retain its current status as "a place to be" for many years to come.

- **Begin at the American Visionary Art Museum (AVAM). This attraction intersects with sites within Walk 4: Inner Harbor Promenade. See Walk 4 for more information on the AVAM.**

- **Covington St. runs behind the museum. Covington was named in honor of Fort Covington, an important site in the repulse of the British during the Battle of Baltimore. Head through the wonderful art in AVAM's courtyard and outbuildings, and then pick up Covington heading uphill.**

- **The second block beyond Federal Hill is E. Cross St., where you'll see Digital Harbor High School. Take a right there. Just a few hundred feet to the right, at 454 Cross, is the Sailor's Union Bethel Methodist Church. It was built in 1873 and was originally** known as the Ship Church. A few decades earlier, a group of sailors led by Captain Samuel Kramer held services on the hull of a wrecked ship anchored near Light St. Eventually, the men raised enough money to buy the building on Cross St. and convert it into a church.

● Continue up E. Cross, passing tidy brick row homes, to the intersection with Riverside Ave. Take a quick detour right on Riverside to #1124. Its variation from all the other houses around you will be immediately evident. This house was originally built as two adjoining houses and stands at one and a half stories (and more than 200 years old). Such houses were originally known as half or alley houses, which were only one room deep. New immigrants and freed slaves usually inhabited these places. Often, their bosses lived nearby and the houses had livery stables behind them.

● Return to E. Cross St. and take a right. When you arrive at the intersection of Cross and Light St., you'll see across the street the wonderful Cross Street Market, still a local favorite. The market began in 1842 and to this day offers tons of vendors selling terrific fresh foods: meat, produce, flowers, and, of course, seafood. The blocks near the market comprise the edge of Federal Hill's business district. Myriad shops and restaurants abound; this is a good place to come hungry. For a pretty comprehensive list of offerings, as well as the lowdown on the annual Federal Hill Festival, visit historicfederalhill.org

● With Cross Street Market in front of you, head north (right) on Light St. Just up on the left is the Blue Agave Restaurant in what used to be the McHenry Theatre—you'll see the name chiseled in the stone above the arched window. The theater operated as a movie house between 1917 and 1971. Continue heading north on Light St.

● When you come to the intersection with Warren Ave., take a right. Warren was named in honor of Dr. Joseph Warren, a Boston patriot who died at Bunker Hill. It was Warren who, in 1775, sent Paul Revere off on his famous ride. The brick row houses in the 300 and 400 blocks of Warren were built in the first years of the 1900s, while the houses between 402 and 413 Warren were built in the 1880s for ship owners.

● Warren Ave. ends here at a little path heading left into the park. Before you take it, take a quick right down this diminutive section of Henry St., paved with Belgian block. Henry St. was also named for a Revolutionary War hero, John Henry. He served in the Continental Congress and was Maryland's first senator. Henry St. soon ends at E. Hamburg St. Most houses on Hamburg were built in the 1830s and 1840s by Baltimore banker John Gittings, whose name lends itself not only to a street two blocks south but also to Gittings Ave. straddling the city/county line (see Walk 33).

● On E. Hamburg, turn right to see the house at #337. It was built in 1810, making it one of Federal Hill's older homes. It served as the headquarters for Union Army General Benjamin F. Butler during the Civil War. Several Confederate spies were held prisoner and then executed at this house. Butler stood on the porch to watch their execution in the courtyard below.

● Return to Henry St. and go straight into Federal Hill Park for one of the best views anywhere. High up on Federal Hill, the Inner Harbor and much of the city beyond opens up in front of you. At the far end of the park, your view follows Federal Hill as it winds toward M&T Bank Stadium, home of the Ravens. At the edge of the hill itself, standing before the harbor, you'll see antique cannons, the 15-star American flag, and the monuments to Colonel George Armistead, commander of Fort McHenry during the Battle of Baltimore in the War of 1812, and Major General Samuel Smith, who served in both the Revolutionary War and the War of 1812, in which he commanded the Third Division of the Maryland Militia during the Battle of Baltimore. (See "Back Story" on page 20 for more on Federal Hill.) On the other side of the park, beyond the swing sets, stands another memorial: the "Our Fathers Saved" sundial, dedicated in 1933 in honor of Union Civil War casualties, a perhaps begrudging honor

Federal Hill row houses

considering Union soldiers had their guns at the ready on a hostile Baltimore citizenry and set up camps along Warren Ave. during an occupation that lasted even longer than the one in New Orleans.

● Head to the northwest end of the park, with Ravens Stadium more or less straight ahead of you, and descend the steps to E. Montgomery St. The street was named for John Montgomery, mayor of Baltimore from 1820 to 1822. It was this road that General Benjamin Butler traveled on his way up Federal Hill during the seizure of Baltimore during the Civil War. This lovely cobblestone block contains some beautiful houses, some dating back to the earliest years of the 19th century. Check out the house at #200½, which holds the distinction of being Baltimore's narrowest house at just over 7 feet wide. The house dates to the middle of the 19th century. The story goes that the original owner lived next door at #200 and tore out a rose garden next to his house so that his grown daughter could live in the new construction.

● Continue heading west on E. Montgomery to #130, a wooden house surviving from circa 1775, before fire mandates required houses to be built of brick. Almost directly across the street, the 1885 three-story brick-front building at #125 once served as the headquarters of the Watchman Fire Company (it does indeed look like a firehouse). In the days before the city took over firefighting duties, individual insurance companies employed their own firefighting forces, the Watchman being one of them. The company was instituted in 1840 and had an earlier office on Light St. Watchman, like the other insurance fire companies, made a habit of rushing to fires to first check to see if the burning building was associated with their company. If not, they waited for the proper company's firefighters to show up.

● You'll soon see a still-functioning fire station as you continue west and reach the intersection with Light St. to the left. This station houses Engine Company 2 and was established in 1920.

● Cross Light St. and continue on Montgomery. The lovely house at #36, built in 1795, is the first house in Federal Hill to have been built of brick. The doorway is a replica; the original, a magnificent work of art, is now in the Baltimore Museum of Art.

● On the right side of the street, #2–12 are 1848 Greek Revival homes. On the left side, #1–11 were built between 1800 and 1810. Around the corner, at 801 S. Charles St., is the Scarborough Faire, built in 1801 and operating today as a B&B.

● E. Montgomery turns to W. Montgomery at Charles St. The neighborhood to the west is the historic African American enclave of Sharp-Leadenhall, which traces its beginnings to 1790, when a small group of free blacks settled here. In the 20th century, the city purchased many original homes through eminent domain and demolished most of them. Those remaining were then sold for one dollar to anyone willing to move in and rehab them. The much-heralded program saved quite a few historic homes that still stand today. However, many of Sharp-Leadenhall's original inhabitants, some with family roots stretching back to the 18th century, were priced out. It's probably worth your time to poke around this neighborhood, but to stay on the Federal Hill tour, turn left at S. Charles St. If you are in need of some refueling, there are plenty of shops and restaurants between here and Cross St., six blocks south.

● Take your second left onto E. Henrietta St. and follow it to the intersection with Light St. Slightly diagonally straight ahead is Warren Ave. Take it. Just ahead on the right is the unique Lee Street Baptist Church, founded in a South Baltimore stable in 1854. (The name of the church today is The Church on Warren Avenue at Federal Hill, more accurately reflecting its current location.) From the outside, you can see the enormous leaded stained glass windows.

● Take a left at the next block, William St., named for Otho Holland Williams, a Revolutionary War colonel. On the next block, at the northwest corner of William and E. Churchill St., is the beautiful brick building that once served as the South Baltimore Station of the Methodist Church. This Classical Revival building dates to 1851 and is now a residential building. Here you can take the narrow Churchill one block east, passing more lovely 19th-century row homes. You won't be surprised to know that this street was originally called Sugar Alley, as its width makes the moniker "alley" more suitable than "street." Churchill will end at Battery Ave. Look just to the right on Battery, at #896, to see a rather wide-front brick house. This is rare as houses were taxed based on sidewalk frontage. Most wealthy homeowners built up instead of out.

Back Story

In 1608, the famed English explorer John Smith came up the Patapsco and sighted "a great red bank of clay flanking a natural harbor basin." For the next 180 years, this hill was known as John Smith's Hill. But then a drunken party of about 4,000 people congregated here in 1788 to celebrate the ratification of the U.S. Constitution by the State of Maryland. The party featured a model sailing ship, the *Federalist*. Men lugged the ship up the hill (and then it subsequently slid down the hill); this, in combination with the ratification of the federal Constitution, meant that the name of the place thereafter was Federal Hill. In 1795 Captain David Porter erected a marine observatory and signal tower on the hill, a perfect vantage point for spotting incoming ships making their way up the Patapsco. For many years thereafter, Federal Hill was also known as Signal Hill. The observatory ceased operation in 1899. Famously, during the Civil War, Union troops fortified Federal Hill and trained their guns on the city. The site officially became a park in 1880 and has continued to grow in popularity as a place for relaxation and recreation.

Directly in front of this house is Federal Hill Park, with the AVAM down the hill on the other side.

POINTS OF INTEREST (START TO FINISH)

American Visionary Art Museum avam.org, 800 Key Hwy., 410-244-1900

Sailor's Union Bethel Methodist Church 454 E. Cross St.

Cross Street Market Cross St. between Light and Charles Sts.

Blue Agave blueagaverestaurant.com, 1032 Light St., 410-576-3938

The Church on Warren Avenue at Federal Hill thechurchonwarrenavenue.com, 113 Warren Ave.

Federal Hill Park Battery Ave. and Warren Ave.

rouTe summary

1. Start at the American Visionary Art Museum on Key Hwy.
2. Go behind the museum and turn left onto Covington St.
3. Turn right onto E. Cross St.
4. Go to #1124 Riverside Ave.
5. Return to Cross St. and take a right.
6. Take a right onto Light St.
7. Take a right onto Warren Ave.
8. Take a right onto Henry St.
9. Take a right onto E. Hamburg St.
10. Return to Henry St. and enter Federal Hill Park.
11. Exit Federal Hill Park at E. Montgomery St. and head west.
12. Take a left onto S. Charles St.
13. Take a left onto E. Henrietta St.
14. Cross Light St. to Warren Ave.
15. Take a left onto William St.
16. Take a right onto E. Churchill St. to Battery Ave./ Federal Hill Park.

CONNeCTING THe WaLKS

As noted above, Walk 4 intersects at the American Visionary Art Museum, the beginning of this walk.

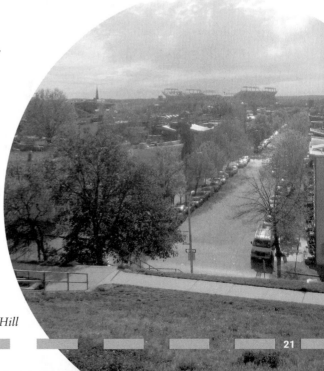

Ravens Stadium from Federal Hill

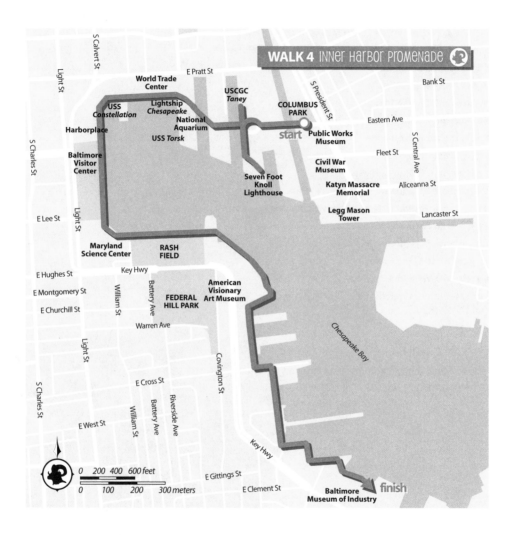

WALK 4 Inner Harbor Promenade

Light St

S Calvert St

E Pratt St

World Trade Center

USCGC *Taney*

Bank St

USS *Constellation*

Lightship *Chesapeake*

COLUMBUS PARK

S President St

Harborplace

National Aquarium

start

Public Works Museum

Eastern Ave

S Central Ave

USS *Torsk*

Fleet St

S Charles St

Baltimore Visitor Center

Civil War Museum

Seven Foot Knoll Lighthouse

Katyn Massacre Memorial

Aliceanna St

Light St

E Lee St

Legg Mason Tower

Lancaster St

Maryland Science Center

RASH FIELD

E Hughes St

Key Hwy

E Montgomery St

Battery Ave

William St

American Visionary Art Museum

E Churchill St

FEDERAL HILL PARK

Warren Ave

Chesapeake Bay

Light St

Covington St

E Cross St

Battery Ave

William St

Riverside Ave

S Charles St

E West St

Key Hwy

0 200 400 600 feet

0 100 200 300 meters

E Gittings St

E Clement St

Baltimore Museum of Industry

finish

4 Inner Harbor Promenade: Tourist Mecca

BOUNDARIES: **Eastern Ave., Inner Harbor Promenade, Key Hwy.**
DISTANCE: **1.9 miles one way**
DIFFICULTY: **Easy to moderate**
PARKING: **Public parking garages in Little Italy near Columbus Park; limited street parking in Harbor East**
PUBLIC TRANSIT: **Water taxi stops in and around the harbor: at the Aquarium, Harborplace, the Science Center, the Rusty Scupper restaurant, Pier Five, and Harbor East. Metro stop at Shot Tower/Marketplace. Both the Charm City Circulator Green and Orange Routes run near the harbor. MTA buses #s 7, 10, 11, and 30 run along Pratt St. MTA bus #64 runs along Light St.**

Baltimore sees some 11 million visitors each year; they are an important economic driver for the city, spending some $3 billion annually. As this book demonstrates, there are a ton of things to do in Charm City, and loads of interesting places to see. But the reality is that the vast majority of visitors to Baltimore head straight for the Inner Harbor and spend the majority of their time there. That's a shame only if they fail to see any more of the city. But lingering in and around the harbor makes sense; it is the city's major draw, hosting a wealth of attractions and putting on Baltimore's best commercial face. Locals sometimes shun the glittering waterside jewel; after all, diehards usually find Baltimore's seedier side the real attraction. And so the snide will scoff at this section as something not real, as a place for the out-of-towners. But even the most obdurate fan of grit and grime will find it almost impossible not to concede that a stroll around the harbor on a day with beautiful weather is a simple pleasure that's hard to beat.

● Start in Columbus Park, which is complete with a series of Italian flags and a beautiful statue of Christopher Columbus, the youngest of the three monuments to Columbus in Baltimore (after Herring Park's 1792 statue and Druid Hill's 1892 memorial). This marble memorial was dedicated in 1984 by Mayor William Donald Schaefer and President Ronald Reagan. It's an impressive statue, and its home in Columbus Piazza is impressive, too. The six reliefs that circle the marble base depict the *Nina,* the *Pinta,* the *Santa Maria,* Genoa, Columbus's landing, and his first meeting with American Indians.

● Head toward the water over the bridge with the old Baltimore Public Works Museum (see Walk 5: Harbor East) to your left onto Pier 5, home to several attractions. The Institute of Marine and Environmental Technology (IMET) is in the old Columbus Center building on the right. IMET is a joint research center involving the University of Maryland, Baltimore County (UMBC); the University of Maryland Center for Environmental Science (UMCES); and the University of Maryland, Baltimore (UMB). The scientists at IMET conduct marine and environmental research.

Floating in the water just in front of the marine research center is the U.S. Coast Guard Cutter *Taney,* named for Supreme Court Chief Justice Roger Taney, a Marylander. The ship enjoyed an illustrious military career but derives its fame today primarily from its distinction as being the last ship still afloat that was involved in the Battle of Pearl Harbor. The *Taney* served in both WWII theaters and helped in the search for Amelia Earhart, among other distinctions. She was decommissioned in 1986 and was added to the National Register of Historic Places two years later. The *Taney* is today part of the collection of the Historic Ships in Baltimore, a maritime museum offering tours of three ships, all National Historic Landmarks, and two light-houses in and around the harbor. (See "Points of Interest" below for more info.)

On the same pier as the *Taney* is the Seven Foot Knoll Lighthouse. The lighthouse was originally built in 1854–1855 and is an example of a screw-pile lighthouse, a distinctive hexagonal building that stands on piles screwed into muddy or sandy river bottoms. The bay once housed many of them. Seven Foot Knoll originally stood at the mouth of the Patapsco but was moved to its present location on Pier 5 in 1988 and was placed on the National Register the following year. The U.S. Coast Guard ran it for many years, employing three rotating lightkeepers who manned the lights and sounded fog warnings.

● Cross the next bridge, passing the impressive Power Plant building, listed on the National Register in 1987. Its large guitar, heralding the Hard Rock Café inside and attached to a tall smokestack, is a distinctive feature. The building itself was con-structed in the first decade of the 20th century and is neoclassical in design. The plant's original function was to supply power to the city's system of electric railways. Later, Baltimore Gas & Electric's predecessor company used it as a central steam-supply plant. Today, there are quite a few shops in this building worth checking out.

With the National Aquarium in front of you, cross the next bridge. The National Aquarium in Baltimore is often cited as the key ingredient in Baltimore's harbor renaissance. To this day, it remains one of the world's truly great aquariums, seeing some 1.5 million visitors annually. Plans for the aquarium began in 1976, when the very notion of a revitalized Inner Harbor, then still a grimy shadow of its old working self—packed wharves mostly—was still a very risky proposition. But because of its position on the harbor and the fact that it consistently ranks as Baltimore's top tourist attraction, the gamble has paid off. (There were some nervous moments, however: see "Back Story" on page 28.)

Docked in front of the aquarium astride Pier 3 are two more historic ships: the Lightship 116 *Chesapeake* and the USS *Torsk* submarine (can't miss that fearsome painted toothy smile). The *Chesapeake* was originally built in Charleston, South Carolina, in 1930. In World War II, she served as a guard vessel off Cape Cod, protecting the port of Boston. Lightships had become obsolete by the 1960s, as they were being replaced by automated light towers. The *Chesapeake* served one more tour of duty in Delaware Bay before being decommissioned in 1971. She then came under the aegis of the National Park Service and was loaned to the city of Baltimore in 1982, when she became part of the Historic Ships in Baltimore. The *Torsk,* built at the Portsmouth Naval Shipyard, was commissioned in 1944 and immediately saw action in the Pacific theater in World War II. The *Torsk* continued work throughout the 1950s and 1960s; she was decommissioned in 1968, recording well in excess of 10,000 dives, and has made her home in Baltimore since 1972.

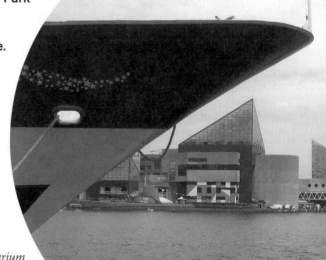

The National Aquarium

- Continue heading west, with the water to your left along the Harbor Promenade. You'll soon pass the 9/11 Monument, appropriately placed in the shadow of Baltimore's World Trade Center. The memorial is constructed of three steel beams from the felled twin towers melded with pieces of limestone from the Pentagon's west wall. Sixty-eight Marylanders lost their lives on September 11, 2001. Baltimore's World Trade Center holds the distinction of being the world's tallest pentagonal building. Enjoy sweeping views of Baltimore from the observation deck on the 27th floor, and take a paddleboat out into the harbor from the promenade in front of the WTC.

- Heading along the water, next up to your right is the Pratt Street Pavilion, one of two major waterside collections of shops and restaurants, all essential in Baltimore's late-20th-century renaissance. A century or two earlier, what you would have seen here were oyster fleets, docks, and wharves, jam-packed with men making a trade in the Chesapeake's bounty. Behind the Pratt Street Pavilion is the USS *Constellation,* truly a magnificent ship with an extraordinary history.

  Ships named *Constellation* hold an illustrious place in American naval history; three have held the name, including today's still-active aircraft carrier known as America's Flagship. The original frigate *Constellation* (1797) was named after the flag of the Continental Congress and became known as the Yankee Racehorse for her extraordinary speed. This is, in essence, what you see in front of you, though the ship underwent major modifications before being restored to her original appearance. A visit on deck never fails to spark the imagination. Her age and significance in American history make her special, but so does the fact that she's a native, built right here in the Sterrett Shipyard. Before the 1700s were over, the *Constellation* had served admirably against the French in the West Indies. She then aided in the blockade of Tripoli in 1802, an event immortalized in the Marine Corps Hymn. Her next service was against the British in the War of 1812 before heading back to service in North Africa. Over the next two decades, the *Constellation* was used in protective services in South America, Asia, the West Indies, North America, and Europe. More global circumnavigations followed before the original *Constellation* was broken up in the 1850s. She was then reborn as a sloop of war in 1854–55. The *Constellation*'s service thereafter was no less extraordinary, including work during the Civil War. The ship today has been beautifully restored to her 1797 appearance with terrific attention to detail. She is truly a delight to visit and absolutely not to be missed.

● Wrap around the open space between the Pratt Street Pavilion and the next complex, the Light Street Pavilion, another collection of shops and restaurants. The space between the two provides an outdoor stage for a variety of public performances, which are often quite good, making it worth a stop to check out whatever's going on.

● Beyond the Light Street Pavilion, at the westward cut for E. Conway St., is Bicentennial Plaza, anchored now with the statue of William Donald Schaefer, the Maryland governor and Baltimore mayor (1971–1987) whose visionary views of the harbor made it what it is today. His bronze likeness (2009) stares out over his great creation, his arm outstretched as if waving to all the passersby—and there are many of them—taking advantage of this wonderful public space.

● Up E. Conway, you'll have an unobstructed view of Oriole Park at Camden Yards, still widely regarded as one of the, if not the, nicest stadiums in Major League Baseball. Next up is the visually striking Baltimore Visitor Center, which complements the nautical theme built into the architecture of the Columbus Center and the Aquarium. Step inside to see what's going on.

● There's more open space on the right, often filled with families on nice days, with the occasional free public concert. Next up, as the harbor makes an eastward swing, is the popular Maryland Science Center, instantly recognizable by the massive tyrannosaurus in the window. Along with the Aquarium, the Science Center is one of the city's top attractions and one of the East Coast's best museums for children.

● Continuing around the harbor, you'll pass an old-style carousel, still operating at more than 100 years old (it was built in 1905). Then comes Rash Field, which has at times hosted an ice rink, sand pits for beach volleyball, and a trapeze school. Current plans are to convert Rash Field to a waterfront park.

● Walk south away from the water and cross Key Hwy. to visit the incomparable American Visionary Art Museum (AVAM). Each spring, AVAM sponsors the wild and incredible Kinetic Sculpture Race, starting from more or less this spot on Key Hwy. and traveling 15 miles around the city, culminating in the water entry in Canton. Participating sculptures can be as small as one single bike—decked out in lunacy, of course—or massive things, some more than 50 feet long. Inevitably, the crowd-pleaser, Fifi the colossal

Back Story

With the benefit of hindsight, the National Aquarium in Baltimore seems a no-brainer. But when Mayor Willie Don Schaefer first pursued the idea in the mid-1970s, it seemed a risky, even impossible, dream. The harbor was still a rather decrepit place, and for a city that needed its public funds for any number of social ills, passing a bond referendum putting the city on the hook for most of the money for its construction, more than $20 million, seemed down-right crazy. But crazy works in Baltimore.

The mayor made his pitch. The citizens approved the bond, and by 1981, the aquarium was built. There had been some trepidation over whether it would come in on time. Schaefer vowed it would or else he'd take a dip in the aquarium's outdoor seal pool. When the schedule lagged, Mayor Schaefer made good on his promise and wore an 1890s-style bathing suit and a straw hat. Clutching an inflatable Donald Duck and accompanied by a live mermaid, Schaefer took his promised dip.

pink poodle, will appear. The museum itself is a true treasure, called by CNN "one of the most fantastic museums anywhere in America." It's true; the place is awesome. But many people aren't even sure what visionary art is. From the museum's website, "Visionary art as defined for the purposes of the American Visionary Art Museum refers to art produced by self-taught individuals, usually without formal training, whose works arise from an innate personal vision that revels foremost in the creative act itself." While that might sound like a recipe for mediocrity, the results in this wild museum are guaranteed to blow you away.

- Across Key Hwy. from the AVAM are the Ritz-Carlton residences, tony places out on the water that count among their residents novelist Tom Clancy. Despite the exclusive address, the promenade winds its way around and through the complex, and you can walk it. That said, the walkway begins to break up in pieces here and there after the Ritz-Carlton (though plans are afoot to complete it so that it stretches all the way to Fort McHenry). Nevertheless, if you're up for one more museum, in a little less than half a mile along the water is the unique Baltimore Museum of Industry, where the goal is to "Relive the Industrial Revolution." Here you can learn about some of the many industrial firsts in Baltimore: the country's first gas company, first disposable bottle cap, first typesetting machine, invention of modern radar, and much more. Just outside the museum is docked the country's only operating steam tugboat.

● **From here, retrace your steps back to your starting point or grab public transport.**

POINTS OF INTEREST (START TO FINISH)

Historic Ships in Baltimore historicships.org; Pier I, 301 E. Pratt St.; 410-539-1797
> USS *Constellation*: historicships.org/constellation; **USCGC** *Taney*: historicships.org/taney; USS *Torsk*: historicships.org/torsk; **LV116** *Chesapeake*: historicships.org/chesapeake; **Seven Foot Knoll Lighthouse**: historicships.org/knoll-lighthouse

National Aquarium in Baltimore aqua.org, 501 E. Pratt St., 410-576-3800

Top of the World Observation Level viewbaltimore.org, 401 E. Pratt St., 27th floor, 410-837-VIEW

Maryland Science Center mdsci.org, 601 Light St., 410-685-5225

Baltimore Visitor Center baltimore.org, 401 Light St., 877-BALTIMORE

American Visionary Art Museum avam.org, 800 Key Hwy., 410-244-1900

Baltimore Museum of Industry thebmi.org, 1415 Key Hwy., 410-727-4808

ROUTE SUMMARY

1. Start at Columbus Park.
2. Head west from Eastern Ave. and cross the water to Pier 5.
3. Cross the bridge to Pier 3.
4. Cross the bridge to Pier 4.
5. Follow the harbor promenade westward around the water.
6. Cross Key Hwy. to the American Visionary Art Museum.
7. Cross Key Hwy. to the Ritz-Carlton.
8. Follow the harbor promenade to the Museum of Industry.

CONNECTING THE WALKS

Several options here. The walk's beginning can easily link up with two walks: Walk 5: Harbor East and Walk 11: Civil War Trail. From the American Visionary Art Museum, you can climb the hill behind you to link up with Walk 3: Federal Hill.

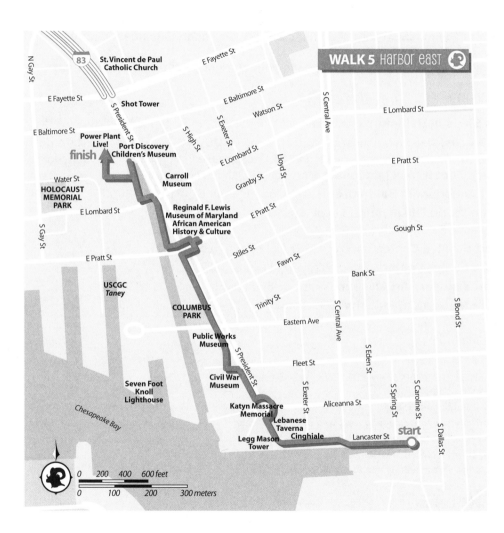

N Gay St

83

St. Vincent de Paul
Catholic Church

E Fayette St

E Fayette St

Shot Tower

E Baltimore St

S President St

Watson St

E Baltimore St

Power Plant
Live!

Port Discovery
Children's Museum

finish

S High St

S Exeter St

E Lombard St

E Lombard St

S Central Ave

E Lombard St

E Pratt St

Water St

Carroll
Museum

Granby St

Lloyd St

E Pratt St

HOLOCAUST
MEMORIAL
PARK

E Lombard St

Reginald F. Lewis
Museum of Maryland
African American
History & Culture

E Pratt St

Gough St

S Gay St

E Pratt St

Stiles St

Fawn St

Bank St

USCGC
Taney

Trinity St

S Bond St

COLUMBUS
PARK

Eastern Ave

S Central Ave

Public Works
Museum

S President St

Fleet St

S Eden St

Civil War
Museum

Seven Foot
Knoll
Lighthouse

S Exeter St

Aliceanna St

S Spring St

S Caroline St

Chesapeake Bay

Katyn Massacre
Memorial

Lebanese
Taverna

Cinghiale

Lancaster St

start

S Dallas St

Legg Mason
Tower

0   200   400   600 feet

0   100   200   300 meters

5 Harbor East: Baltimore's New Half-Billion-Dollar Jewel

BOUNDARIES: **S. Caroline St., Lancaster St., S. President St.**
DISTANCE: **1 mile one way**
DIFFICULTY: **Easy**
PARKING: **Street and garage parking available on S. Caroline St.**
PUBLIC TRANSIT: **Shot Tower Metro Station; both the Charm City Circulator Green and Orange Routes and the Harbor East Shuttle run through Harbor East.**

Harbor East is the city's newest and hippest destination, a natural and long overdue adjunct to the Inner Harbor, just to the west. The half-billion-dollar construction explosion in Harbor East over the past decade has been nothing short of amazing. At a time when so many city centers around the country are full of stalled construction projects because of the economic downturn, and at a time when suburban sprawl continues to chew up open space, it's wonderful to see so much mixed-use, environmentally conscious city-center construction.

● Begin at S. Caroline St., named for the sister of Frederick Calvert, the last Lord of Baltimore. You're just beyond the western edge of Fells Point, in an area that was a sort of no-man's-land until recent years. This is the beginning of what people used to refer to as Inner Harbor East but is now known simply as Harbor East. You'll see the continued building boom along the water here as you head north along S. Caroline St. At the first major block, take a left onto Lancaster St. and follow the brick promenade as it skirts the edge of the water. All of these major new buildings to your right along Lancaster St. have been built since the beginning of the new millennium, starting with the apartment complex just as you turned from S. Caroline St.

● As you continue along Lancaster St., you'll see why this area has been primed for a building explosion for years. Sitting right on the harbor and a stone's throw from downtown and Fells Point, all these buildings mix residential and commercial for terrific city living. Looming ahead of you is the unmistakable Legg Mason Tower, a 24-story, 660,000-square-foot glass and steel edifice. Just before you reach the Legg Mason Tower, check out the Lebanese Taverna, on the corner of Lancaster St. and S. President St., for some terrific Lebanese food.

● Follow S. President St. as it picks up where Lancaster St. ends and moves to the right of the Legg Mason Tower. More new buildings flank the road, including the Spinnaker Bay luxury apartments, which also house several ground-floor businesses, including acclaimed Italian restaurant Cinghiale, noted for its terrific food and extensive wine list. Straight ahead is a cobblestone traffic circle with the arresting 40-foot-tall Katyn Massacre Memorial (dedicated in 2000) in the middle, strikingly designed to commemorate the massacre of 22,000 Polish prisoners by the Soviet Union in WWII.

Every spoke of this traffic wheel offers more of something—down International Dr., to the left, for example, is the new Four Seasons Hotel. Down Aliceanna St. to the left, you'll find more easy access to the harbor, with more restaurants, shopping, a new Marriott hotel, and a marina. On the right after Spinnaker Bay is a fitness center and a seven-screen Landmark movie theater. While a movie theater might not seem such an essential part of urban living, its presence definitely filled a void downtown. One thing that is essential to urban living is access to groceries; one block east of where you are on S. President St., to the right on Fleet St., is Whole Foods Market. Beyond the circle on S. President St., on your left, is one of the finest Irish pubs around, James Joyce.

● Continue moving north along S. President St. to #601, the President Street Station, just before you reach Fleet St. While everything to the immediate south is virtually brand spanking new, this little old building survives for at least one very important reason: the first casualties of the Civil War occurred here, on April 19, 1861. Eventually, more than 600,000 Americans died in the Civil War, but the first 16 perished in the blocks near the station, where a Southern-sympathizing mob attacked a Massachusetts regiment sent through President Street Station on the way to defend Washington, D.C. When the clash was over, 5 soldiers and at least 11 civilians lay dead. Baltimorean Catherine Smith wrote of the event at the time, "[There] was one battle from the President Street Depot . . . A good deal of blood was spilled on both sides." (For more on this battle and its aftermath, see Walk 11: Civil War Trail.) Even without this attendant history, the President Street Station holds an important place in American history: built in 1849, it remains the country's oldest major city railroad terminal. Go inside to check it out; the station today is home to the Baltimore Civil War Museum, now reopened after closure due to city budget cuts and run now by the Maryland Historical Society (MHS). This is a wonderful arrangement, as not only has the building remained open, but also its displays and the stories it can tell relating to slavery, abolitionism, railroading, and the Civil War are far-reaching due to the MHS's extensive collections.

- Continue north on S. President St. to the extraordinary brick building on your left, just before Eastern Ave. This 1912 still-functioning pumping station was once the home of the fascinating Public Works Museum. When it operated, it was apparently the only public works museum in the world: a massive museum dedicated to sewers, water treatment, and the maze of plumbing operations that exist under the city streets, including a rare 1780s wooden drain pipe. But, like the City Life Museums, Public Works became a victim of shrinking city budgets; hopefully, it will be resurrected when times are more flush.

- Continue walking north along S. President St. To the left at E. Falls Ave. and Eastern Ave. is Columbus Park, complete with a series of Italian flags and a beautiful statue of Christopher Columbus, the youngest of the three monuments to Columbus in Baltimore (after Herring Park's 1792 statue and Druid Hill's 1892 memorial).

- Continue north along S. President St. for another couple of blocks and cross S. President at E. Pratt St. to the first building on the corner, at 830 E. Pratt. This is the Reginald F. Lewis Museum of Maryland African American History & Culture, which opened in 2005. This is a wonderful addition to Baltimore's museum scene and an overdue nod to the essential role African Americans have played in the shaping of Maryland and the United States. The museum is affiliated with the Smithsonian Institution and is the largest African American museum on the East Coast. The experience begins even before you walk through the door; the building itself is an arresting presence, with bold colors and intersecting lines and angles. Inside, the museum tells the story of centuries of African American experience in Maryland with an incredible collection of artifacts, rare books, art, music, and many other items.

- After visiting the Reginald F. Lewis Museum, cross S. President St. again at E. Pratt St. and take an immediate right so that you're paralleling the canal of the Jones Falls. (If you haven't eaten yet, consider Miss Shirley's Café on the corner, a Baltimore institution that has garnered some national attention.) This is a lovely spot: To the north you'll see the prominent Shot Tower and the bell tower of St. Vincent de Paul Catholic Church (see Walk 10: Little Italy & Jonestown/Old Town); to the east is the Carroll

Museum and Little Italy; to the south your eye will follow the ribbon of the Jones Falls, the city's original dividing line, as it spills into the harbor. To the west is downtown, with its tall buildings and general vibe of commerce and bustle.

● Continue north for another block along S. President St. to the Port Discovery Children's Museum. If you don't have little ones with you and thus have little interest in entering the Children's Museum, at least take a few moments to admire the lovely brick building that houses it. This is the Fish Market building, built in 1907. This area originally housed one of the city's main markets, established in 1787, along with Fells Point and Lexington Markets. But the area was destroyed in the Great Fire of 1904, and the Fish Market building represents the first stabs at rebuilding. Look for two nearby markers: the 1904 Fire Remembrance marker on the outside of the west wall of the building and the Centre Market commission marker, commemorating the rebuilding of the area after the fire. Both sit near the Booth Fountain, donated by businessman Alfred Booth in 1906 to mark the rapid reconstruction of Baltimore's downtown.

● Behind the Port Discovery Children's Museum is Power Plant Live!. To go there, use the Water St. entrance, to the left of the museum if you are facing the entrance. This area has become one of the city's hot spots for entertainment and nightlife, with restaurants, bars, nightclubs, and Rams Head Live, which hosts many national touring acts. From May through October, Power Plant Live! offers free public music in the plaza.

● At 608 Water St., in the old Chocolate Factory building, you can check out Baltimore's newest museum as of January 2012: the National Pinball Museum. Yes, it's exactly what it sounds like: the history and cultural impact of pinball, plus the opportunity to try your hand on some machines. More than 100, both new and vintage, are on display.

● You are just a couple of blocks north of the Inner Harbor and Baltimore's tourist mecca. It's easy to retrace your steps to where you began this walk, but there are a thousand other options here. For another walk, see "Connecting the Walks," opposite page.

POINTS OF INTEREST (START TO FINISH)

Lebanese Taverna lebanesetaverna.com, 719 S. President St., 410-244-5533

Cinghiale cgeno.com, 822 Lancaster St., 410-547-8282

Katyn Massacre Memorial katynbaltimore.com, S. President St. roundabout

President Street Station / Baltimore Civil War Museum 601 President St., 443-220-0290

The Reginald F. Lewis Museum of Maryland African American History & Culture 830 E. Pratt St., 443-263-1800

Miss Shirley's Café missshirleys.com, 750 E. Pratt St., 410-528-5373

Port Discovery Children's Museum portdiscovery.org, 35 Market Pl., 410-727-8120

Power Plant Live! powerplantlive.com, 34 Market Pl., 410-752-5483

National Pinball Museum nationalpinballmuseum.org, 608 Water St., 443-438-1241

For more general information about the area and development, visit harboreast.com.

rouTe SuMMary

1. Start at S. Caroline St., between Lancaster St. and Thames St.
2. Turn left onto Lancaster St.
3. Turn right onto S. President St.
4. Cross S. President St. east to visit the Reginald F. Lewis Museum on E. Pratt St.
5. Cross S. President St. west to visit Port Discovery and Power Plant Live!.

CONNeCTING THe WaLKS

Several walks are very close by. Walk 11: Civil War Trail begins at President Street Station. Walk 4: Inner Harbor begins at Columbus Park. Walk 10: Little Italy & Jonestown/Old Town begins on S. Exeter St., three blocks north of Lancaster St.

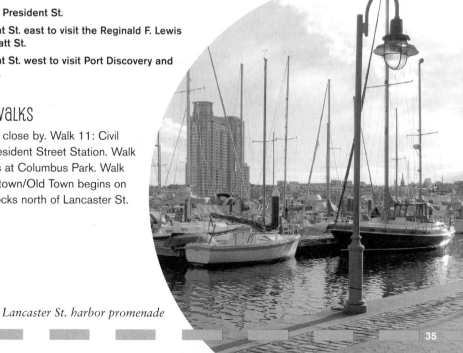

Lancaster St. harbor promenade

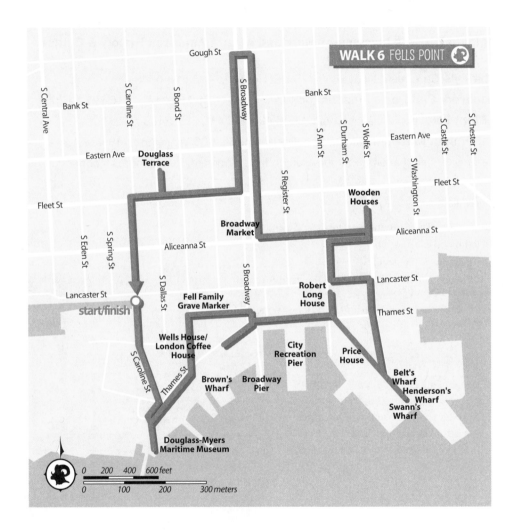

WALK 6 FELLS POINT

Gough St

Bank St

S Central Ave

Bank St

S Caroline St

S Bond St

S Broadway

Eastern Ave

Douglass Terrace

Fleet St

S Register St

Bank St

S Ann St

S Durham St

S Wolfe St

Eastern Ave

S Castle St

S Chester St

S Washington St

Fleet St

Wooden Houses

Broadway Market

Aliceanna St

Aliceanna St

S Eden St

S Spring St

S Dallas St

S Broadway

Lancaster St

Lancaster St

Fell Family Grave Marker

Robert Long House

Thames St

start/finish

Wells House/ London Coffee House

S Caroline St

Thames St

Brown's Wharf

Broadway Pier

City Recreation Pier

Price House

Belt's Wharf

Henderson's Wharf

Swann's Wharf

Douglass-Myers Maritime Museum

0   200   400   600 feet

0   100   200   300 meters

6 FELLS POINT: SEVERAL WORLDS IN ONE

BOUNDARIES: **S. Caroline St., Philpot St., Fell St., S. Wolfe St., Bank St.**
DISTANCE: **2.5 miles**
DIFFICULTY: **Moderate**
PARKING: **Garage and street parking on S. Caroline St., near Lancaster St. Street and meter parking in the heart of Fells Point, but restrictions and many people vying for spots make parking difficult, depending on time of day.**
PUBLIC TRANSIT: **MTA bus #11 runs along Fleet St.; MTA buses #10 and #30 run along Broadway. The water taxi stops at Broadway Pier.**

This part of Baltimore has been around for a while. Yes, Old Town and Jonestown are older, but they would be unrecognizable to a time traveler from the 18th century. Much of Fells Point, on the other hand, looks very much like it did a couple of centuries ago. The entire neighborhood is a National Historic District, with more than 160 individual buildings on the National Register. The Englishman William Fell was a speculator on the prowl for good ship-building land when he made his purchase in 1726, naming it Fell's Prospect. His son Edward began laying out the streets, giving them names that reminded him of the mother country. Eventually, Edward sold off plots of land, and by 1763 the area known as Fells Point was born; it was incorporated into Baltimore-Town in 1773. In addition to that colonial history, Fells Point possesses sites important to Frederick Douglass, for my money one of the most extraordinary humans this country has ever produced. But if all this history and colonial beauty isn't enough for you, Fells Point also happens to have some of Baltimore's best bars and restaurants. And if Latin food is your thing, Upper Fells Point is the place to be. It's little wonder that after the Inner Harbor, Fells Point is probably Baltimore's next stop for out-of-towners. But a walk here also has the power to remind locals why they do (or should) love this city. Every October, more than half a million people descend on the neighborhood for the Fells Point Fun Festival, held annually for almost 50 years now. The Annual Historic Harbor House Tour of Fells Point has been held every Mother's Day for almost as long. It's a great opportunity to see inside some of these colonial beauties. And, of course, there are several commercial ghost tours of Fells Point. Indeed, this neighborhood, with its long history of brothels and bars, is haunted by several ghosts. Fells Point is several worlds in one, all of them a treat.

● Start on S. Caroline St., south of Lancaster St. As you head toward the water, passing the Living Classrooms site, you'll first come across a large open area on your right, just past Dock St. The site extends southward for several blocks, past Philpot St., named for Brian Philpot Jr., who emigrated from England to Baltimore in the mid- to late 1700s. This is the AlliedSignal Site, where, in 1845, Isaac Tyson Jr. founded the country's first bichromate plant. The factory processed chromium until the late 1990s. The site underwent extensive environmental cleanup and awaits reuse. Perhaps it's apocryphal, but some historians believe that the term "hooker" originated on this slice of land, as it was originally shaped like a hook and many prostitutes used to ply their trade here.

In an 1846 speech in England, Frederick Douglass recalled the ghastliness of this area: "Many a night have I been wakened in Philpotts-street, Baltimore, by the passing-by, at midnight, of hundreds of slaves, carrying their chains and fetters and uttering cries and howlings, almost enough to startle the dead. They were going to the market to work in cotton or sugar, going off to be killed in the space of five or six years, in the swamps of Alabama, Georgia, and Louisiana."

● At the end of S. Caroline St., where it intersects with Philpot St., continue heading straight toward the water and you will soon come to the Frederick Douglass–Isaac Myers Maritime Park. This is a unique museum, focusing on the extraordinary lives of its two namesakes. While many recognize Frederick Douglass, Isaac Myers remains a little-known figure. But his life was also astonishing. Myers owned and operated a shipyard, the Chesapeake Marine Railway & Dry Dock Company, just one block west at Philpot and Wills Sts.; he was the first African American in the country to own and run a shipyard. Just outside the front door of the museum is a repair site for historic ships. In between is a bust of Frederick Douglass. Artist Marc Andre Robinson created and installed this striking sculpture in 2006. Douglass's presence here next to the ship repair facility is apropos; during slavery he worked these very docks as a ship caulker. See the "Back Story" on page 40 for more on Douglass.

● Turn around to head back in the direction of S. Caroline St., but take a right onto Thames St. The street's name is meant to mirror London's famous river. If asking directions, however, don't be surprised to hear the name pronounced several different ways: "Thames" with a long "a"; "Tems," like the river; and "Thames" with a soft "th."

(Most Baltimoreans either pronounce it with a hard "T" and long "a" or with a "th" at the top.) In another block, you'll come to Bond St. To your right is the brightly painted Bond St. Wharf, a renovated retail and office space complex.

On the corner of Thames St. and Bond St., at 1532–34 Thames, used to be a house owned by George Wells. He owned and operated a shipyard across the street and received the Continental Congress's commission for the *Virginia,* the first ship of the navy for a country on the brink of a revolution. Wells went on to build many other ships as part of a fleet of shipbuilders throughout Fells Point; many of these ships saw action in the War of 1812. Today, the CanUSA corporation, a paper-recycling company, has its headquarters in this renovated building.

Connected to the Wells House, on the corner at 854 S. Bond St., is the façade of the old London Coffee House (1752), the last surviving colonial-era coffee house in the United States. Here, pre-Revolutionary patriots met to talk about the coming insurrection against the British.

Head north along S. Bond St. Here, as with many other Fells Point streets, you'll notice the beautiful road surfaces. While most casual observers call it cobblestone, it's actually Belgian block. The effect is wonderful, both visually and practically, as it forces automobiles to slow down and makes a pleasing sound. As you walk north, you're getting closer to the 600 block, home of the H&S Bakery. You might catch a whiff of some enticing aromas. (If the smell is too tempting, you can buy breads at H&S's outlet store on 1616 Fleet St.) But for now, take a right before you get to the bakery, onto Shakespeare St., revealing a quintessential Fells Point lane: brick row houses jammed together and

Bond Street Wharf

Back Story

Perhaps more than any other person in this country's history, Frederick Douglass represents the ideals behind what is commonly referred to as the American Dream: that if you work hard enough, you will be rewarded. Douglass's rise and what he accomplished in his life are nothing short of astonishing. Born into slavery on Maryland's Eastern Shore, Douglass was moved to Baltimore as a very young man, a move for which he was grateful, as he stated that city slaves were generally treated better than those in rural areas. Douglass wrote, "Going to live at Baltimore laid the foundation, and opened the gateway, to all my subsequent prosperity. I have ever regarded it as the first plain manifestation of that kind providence which has ever since attended me, and marked my life with so many favors." He lived on Aliceanna St. in Fells Point and worked as a ship caulker. Inviting brutal whippings, Douglass taught himself to read, employing tricks on neighborhood kids and paying poor white kids with bread to teach him. In the end, Douglass rose from illiterate slave to eventually penning several books, earned international fame as an eloquent orator and abolitionist, and achieved the rank of U.S. ambassador to Haiti. He lived long enough to see slavery abolished and pass into the mists of history. But the man always carried the scars. His story and his writings are essential to every American wishing to understand this country.

looking very much like they have for more than two centuries. On this short two-block street lived no fewer than five ship captains, including Captain William Furlong, a successful privateer who lived at #1608. His residence dates to 1796. Across the street, at #1607, is the Fell family grave marker. Four male members of the Fell family are buried here. The block's oldest house is #1600, dating to 1770.

● Continue to the end of Shakespeare St. to where it intersects with S. Broadway. Here you'll emerge onto a plaza lined with shops, bars, and restaurants. To the left, at 806 S. Broadway, is the Vagabond Theatre, home of the Vagabond Players. This theater is the country's oldest continuously operated "little theater," begun in 1916. Its first production was H. L. Mencken's *The Artist*. When F. Scott and Zelda Fitzgerald were living in Baltimore, the Vagabond Players produced her play, *Scandalabra*. Unfortunately, it was a flop. Next door, at #802, is the site of Seaman's Hall, the first local longshoreman's union (1912). The union was later instrumental in the creation of the National Maritime Union, dramatically improving the working conditions and lives of seamen.

- Head south on S. Broadway, toward the water. On the corner of S. Broadway and Thames is the Admiral Fell Inn. The space the inn now occupies at 888 S. Broadway has been hosting visitors, initially seamen on shore leave, for almost 250 years. The inn today consists of seven adjoining buildings, the oldest of which date to the 1770s and 1780s. In 1889, the Woman's Auxiliary of the Port Mission created the Anchorage here, a place where seamen could retire for the night with their Christian consciences intact. The Anchorage's cellars were eventually turned into a vinegar bottling plant, which closed in 1976. The Admiral Fell Inn took over in 1985 and has become one of the finest and most interesting hotels around, garnering charter membership in the National Trust for Historic Hotels of America.

- Continue heading west on Thames St. to check out this largely intact 18th-century row. At 1626 Thames is The Horse You Came In On Saloon, established in 1775. Sometimes visited by Edgar Allan Poe, The Horse is the country's only saloon to have operated before, during, and after Prohibition, making it America's oldest continuously operating saloon. William Fell's mansion stood at #1621, when this street was named Fell's Street. Unfortunately, it was demolished many years ago.

- Across the street is Brown's Wharf, which today houses shops and offices, including Jhpiego, a nonprofit international health organization affiliated with the Johns Hopkins University. But when it was built in 1820, it served as a warehouse for flour and coffee.

- Turn around and head back toward S. Broadway, crossing the plaza. On the water to your right is Broadway Pier. Regular ferry service between here and Locust Point ended in 1937. In the decades prior to that, this same ferry offloaded thousands of newly arrived immigrants just processed at a nearby immigration station. Still an entry point for new immigrants today, Baltimore has a long history of immigration and absorption, evidenced in the eclectic place names and ethnic enclaves scattered throughout the city. For many years in the late 19th and early 20th century, only Ellis Island saw more new arrivals than Baltimore, as many as 40,000 a year. By the close of the 19th century, the vast majority of these immigrants were Polish and Italian.

Next to Broadway is City Recreation Pier, in the 1700 block of Thames St. You might recognize City Recreation Pier as the home of NBC's *Homicide: Life on the Street* (1993–1999), a creation of Barry Levinson and David Simon, both Baltimoreans. Levinson used Fells Point for filming locations in his films *Avalon, Diner, Liberty Heights,* and *Tin Men* as well. Fans of *Homicide* will recognize the bar across the street from City Recreation Pier as the one owned by three homicide cops in the show. In real life, it's the Waterfront Hotel (a bar, not a hotel), housed in a 1771 building, the city's second-oldest brick building. During the Civil War, the Waterfront housed soldiers.

● Continue along Thames St., taking in the colonial character, until you reach the amazing house at #1732. It was built in 1800 and remains in pristine and original condition. This merchant's house is three and a half stories, typical of wealthy merchants' houses. Close by, 1738 Thames St. was originally a tavern, built in the 18th century. It became a clothing sweatshop in the early 20th century.

● When you reach the next block, S. Ann St., take a left for a quick detour to the Robert Long House at 812 S. Ann. This street was named for Ann Fell, Edward Fell's wife. When Edward died, Ann continued selling plots of land; her financial acumen made her one of colonial America's most successful businesswomen. The Robert Long House is the city's oldest existing residence, dating to 1765. Long served as a quartermaster for the Continental Navy. The house is open to visitors, who can see rooms furnished with Revolutionary War period pieces. Today, the house serves as the headquarters of the Society for the Preservation of Federal Hill and Fells Point. The preservation society was an outgrowth of the "Stop the Road" citizen uprising formed to halt the construction of a freeway that would have cut off Fells Point from the water. That's unthinkable today, but in the 1960s, Fells Point had deteriorated into a seedy backwater. In fact, the neighborhood had, almost from the beginning, maintained a reputation as a carnivalesque place. One visitor in 1798 remarked, "Here ships land their cargoes and here the crews wait not even for twilight to fly to the polluted arms of the white, black, and yellow harlot." But in a city that tolerates, even welcomes, the real and shuns artifice, Fells Point had always been a somewhat celebrated seedy backwater. Even in the late 20th century, locals were still celebrating its uniqueness. Indeed, Fells Point serves as the inspiration for several of John Waters's early films, such as *Pink Flamingos, Multiple Maniacs,* and *Polyester.* Fortunately, in the 1960s, a sufficient number of locals were horrified by the prospect of a freeway destroying their neighborhood's character. Led by a then-unknown social worker named Barbara Mikulski, they fought to save the neighborhood. Thank goodness they did. That fight led to the revitalization of the neighborhood and, of course, kickstarted Mikulski's political career. In 2012, she became the longest-serving woman in the history of the United States Congress.

● Turn around and return to Thames St., taking a diagonal left down Fell St. At 910 Fell St., on the right, you will see the William Price house. Price made a fantastic living building Baltimore schooners in the late 1700s. His shipyard was behind the house. Across the street, at #909, is where Price's son, John, also a shipbuilder, lived. Frederick Douglass worked at the Prices' shipyard just before he made his break to freedom. Just up the block from the younger Price's house, at #931, was the home of shipbuilder John Steele. The house was constructed in 1786. Across the street, at #936, is Belt's Wharf, built in 1877 to serve as the port for the fleet of the C. Morton Stewart coffee distributors. Today, it houses condos.

● At the end of the street are two more wharves, Swann's and Henderson's. Swann's Wharf, at 1001 Fell St., is one of the older warehouses in Fells Point, dating to the 1820s. Swann is a locally prominent name; Thomas Swann served as mayor of Baltimore and governor of Maryland, as well as the president of the B&O Railroad. Henderson's Wharf, at Fell and Wolfe Sts., was a disembarkation site for European immigrants before 1850. The

Near Broadway Market

warehouse there, built in 1897, stored tobacco for European export. Today, there is an inn and private residences. Take a moment to enjoy the terrific water views before turning around and heading north on S. Wolfe St.

● Up the block to the right at Wolfe and Thames Sts., across from Thames Street Park, is the National Can Company building, which employed immigrants canning the Chesapeake's bounty for 100 years, between 1880 and 1980. The sheer volume helped to propel Baltimore to its status as the world's largest canning center. The building was converted to apartments in 1983.

● Cross the park and take a left onto Lancaster St. The third house on the left was the home of William Tinker, a local grocer. In the 1700s, this was a two-and-a-half-story dormered house, but it has seen many changes over the years.

● Take your next right onto S. Ann St. Just up the block, to the left, is the Gothic-style St. Stanislaus Kostka Roman Catholic Church. The church was built in 1889 to serve the area's growing Polish community. In 1936 in this church, local longshoremen voted to strike, a bold move and a significant one for organized labor.

● Head north. Take a right onto Aliceanna St., named for Aliceanna Webster Bond, wife of John Bond, who helped settle Fells Point. Your next destination is two blocks away, where you'll take a left onto S. Wolfe St. to the 600 block. But be on the lookout for the historical marker at the corner of the first block, S. Durham St., which gives you the lowdown on Frederick Douglass and the time he spent living here on Aliceanna St.

The houses at 612–614 Wolfe St. are unique. Each is one and a half stories and built of wood, surviving from circa 1775, before fire mandates required houses to be built of brick. Three more wooden houses can be seen on S. Ann St., at #533, #717, and #719. The story behind the name of this street is interesting as well. The Wolfe here is British General James Wolfe, a victorious soldier in a 1759 battle against the French in Canada. That the street name retained its association even after the revolution is rather striking.

● Return to Aliceanna and take a right, following it to S. Broadway. If you didn't before, take some time to poke around the shops here, or head into the terrific Broadway Market, on the right. Broadway Market has been at this location in one form or another since 1786. It was originally known as Fells Point Market and retained that name until 1797, when it became known by its current name. Recent work has refurbished some of the market, making it an even more inviting place to come and get some great food.

● Continue north on S. Broadway to Bank St. (three blocks north). At the corner is St. Patrick's Roman Catholic Church, which is the second-oldest church in the Baltimore diocese, founded in 1792. The current structure is not that old, however; it was built in 1897, replacing the original church building. The locally beloved Cardinal James Gibbons served his first assignment at St. Patrick's, in 1861, before being named a cardinal and pushing for the creation of the Catholic University of America, eventually becoming its first chancellor. The church suffered some minor damage during the freak 5.8-magnitude earthquake Baltimore suffered in 2011.

If you're hungry, this is a great place to be. You're now in the vicinity of what is known as Upper Fells Point, and it's likely that you are hearing more Spanish than English. Many immigrants from Mexico and Central America have settled in this area in recent years. One of the benefits for longtime locals is a plethora of Latin restaurants. You'll find plenty by heading a few blocks north.

● Once you've had your gustatory fill, return south on S. Broadway, back to Fleet St., and take a right. In three blocks, you'll reach S. Dallas St. On this corner, in 1773, you would have seen Baltimore's first Methodist meetinghouse. It's no longer there, but head north on S. Dallas to see Douglass Terrace. When Frederick Douglass returned to Fells Point a half century after his time there as a slave, the then world-famous orator, ambassador, and author built five houses here and named them Douglass Terrace. The houses still stand today.

● Continue north on S. Dallas for a few hundred feet until you reach Eastern Ave. Diagonally to the right is the Baltimore Tattoo Museum, dedicated to the art of tattooing dating back to the 19th century. Because the museum also houses a fully functioning tattoo parlor, you might consider leaving with a more permanent souvenir.

● Return to Fleet St. and take a right. The next block is S. Caroline St. Take a left there. Your starting point is two blocks south.

POINTS OF INTEREST (STALL TO FINISH)

Frederick Douglass–Isaac Myers Maritime Park douglassmyers.org, 1417 Thames St.,
410-685-0295

George Wells House / London Coffee House Northwest corner of Bond and Thames Sts.
/ 854 S. Bond St.

Brown's Wharf Broadway and Thames St.

Fell Family Grave Marker 1607 Shakespeare St.

The Vagabond Theatre vagabondplayers.org, 806 S. Broadway, 410-563-9135

Seaman's Hall 802 S. Broadway

Admiral Fell Inn harbormagic.com, 888 South Broadway, 410-539-2000

The Horse You Came In On thehorsebaltimore.com, 1626 Thames St., 410-327-8111

Broadway Pier Broadway and Thames St.

City Recreation Pier 1700 block of Thames St.

Merchant's House 1732 Thames St.

Tavern / Sweatshop 1738 Thames St.

Robert Long House 812 S. Ann St.

Society for the Preservation of Federal Hill and Fells Point preservationsociety.com,
410-675-6750

Captain John Steele House 931 Fell St.

Belt's Wharf 936 Fell St.

Henderson's Wharf Fell and Wolfe Sts.

Swann's Wharf 1001 Fell St.

William Price House 910 Fell St.

St. Stanislaus Kostka Roman Catholic Church Aliceanna and S. Ann Sts.

Wooden Houses 612–614 Wolfe St.

Broadway Market 600 and 700 blocks of S. Broadway

St. Patrick's Roman Catholic Church Broadway and Bank St.

Douglass Terrace Dallas St.

Baltimore Tattoo Museum baltimoretattoomuseum.net, 1534 Eastern Ave., 410-522-5800

route summary

1. Start at S. Caroline St. and go south to visit the Douglass-Myers Maritime Park.
2. Take a right onto Thames St.
3. Turn left onto S. Bond St.
4. Turn right onto Shakespeare St.
5. See the sites on S. Broadway and then turn right.
6. Turn right onto Thames St.
7. Turn around and head east on Thames St.
8. Take a left onto S. Ann St.
9. Return to Thames St. and take a left onto Fell St.
10. Go north on S. Wolfe St.
11. Take a left onto Lancaster St.
12. Take a right onto S. Ann St.
13. Take a right onto Aliceanna St.
14. Take a left onto S. Wolfe St.
15. Return to Aliceanna St. and take a right.
16. Take a right onto S. Broadway to visit Upper Fells Point.
17. Head south on S. Broadway and take a right onto Fleet St.
18. Turn right onto S. Dallas St.
19. Return to Fleet St. and turn right.
20. Turn left onto S. Caroline St.

connecting the walks

The starting point of this walk is essentially the same starting point (though moving in the opposite direction) of Walk 5: Harbor East.

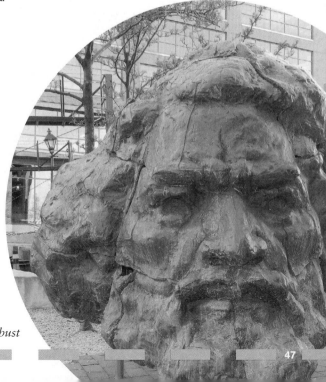

Frederick Douglass bust

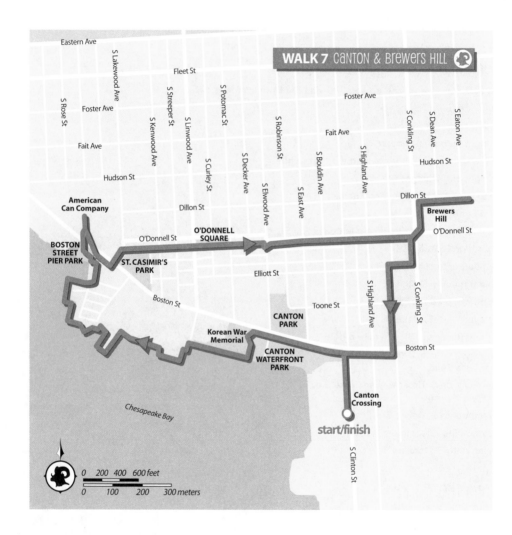

Eastern Ave

S Lakewood Ave

Fleet St

S Rose St

Foster Ave

S Streeper St

S Kenwood Ave

S Linwood Ave

S Potomac St

S Robinson St

Foster Ave

Fait Ave

S Conkling St

S Dean Ave

S Eaton Ave

Fait Ave

Hudson St

S Curley St

S Decker Ave

S Elwood Ave

S Bouldin Ave

S East Ave

S Highland Ave

Hudson St

Hudson St

WALK 7 CaNTON & Brewers Hill

American Can Company

Dillon St

Dillon St

Brewers Hill

BOSTON STREET PIER PARK

O'Donnell St

O'DONNELL SQUARE

O'Donnell St

ST. CASIMIR'S PARK

Elliott St

Boston St

Toone St

S Highland Ave

S Conkling St

CANTON PARK

Korean War Memorial

CANTON WATERFRONT PARK

Boston St

Canton Crossing

Chesapeake Bay

start/finish

S Clinton St

0   200 400 600 feet

0   100   200   300 meters

7 canton & brewers Hill: OLD INDUSTRY and renewed waterfront

BOUNDARIES: **S. Boston St., S. Conkling St., S. Lakewood St., Dillon St., S. Clinton St.**
DISTANCE: **2.5 miles**
DIFFICULTY: **Moderate**
PARKING: **All along route, but free and easy parking can be found at Canton Crossing and the Canton Waterfront Park.**
PUBLIC TRANSIT: **Water Taxi stops at Canton Waterfront Park. MTA buses #s 7, 11, and 13 stop on Clinton St., near Canton Crossing; #11 and #13 run along Boston St.; #7 runs along S. Conkling; and #13 stops on O'Donnell.**

Many locals know Canton primarily as a desirable and safe neighborhood, full of shops and restaurants, new residential construction projects, and an enviable position abutting the northeast section of the Harbor. It is all those things. But Canton also hides an extraordinary history, able to tell some of the more interesting stories in Baltimore's history. Situated east of the original Baltimore-Town and oriented toward the water, Canton was the site in 1797 of the launching of the *Constellation* (see Walk 4) and the creation of the armor plates for the USS *Monitor*. By the 1820s, under the direction of Peter Cooper and Columbus O'Donnell, the son of Canton's founder, John O'Donnell, Canton constituted the country's first large industrial park, a 10,000-acre complex of various manufacturers, fertilizer plants, canners, and bottlers, plus nearby sea lanes and rail lines to export it all. But it wasn't all work; racetracks and beer gardens abounded for recreation. When most of these places disappeared, the US government took over a large swath and created Fort Holabird, where, among other lasting inventions, engineers created army-olive paint, blackout lights, clog-resistant motorcycle fenders, and the US army's inimitable and iconic Willys jeep. Canton today is a great destination, with wonderful residential spots, easy access to the water, and a bevy of watering holes that do its brewing history proud.

● **Begin at the Canton Crossing development off S. Clinton St. The development, anchored by the First Mariner Tower, offers a few restaurants and plenty of street and lot parking.**

Here, on the south corner of Boston St. and Clinton, is where the Potter's Course (1823), a second area racetrack and later known as Kendall Track, was built. It was the site of the 1840 Whig Convention, where Henry Clay and Daniel Webster gave speeches and where William Henry Harrison was nominated for president, giving the occasion the distinction of being the country's first presidential nominating convention. (The Whigs were back four years later, in 1844, when they nominated Henry Clay for the presidency.) Also nearby were the sites of the city's first public bathing beach, as well as a baptismal area where the city's Baptists were dunked into the Patapsco in prodigious numbers, earning the spot the moniker "Baptizing Shore."

● Head north toward Boston St. and go left, more or less following the waterline toward Canton Waterfront Park. To the west, just off Boston St. and S. East St., you'll see the Baltimore City Marine Police Unit building, a small facility where the police unit's marine rescue equipment is stored. Across Boston St. is the Clarence "Du" Burns Arena. Named for the city's first African American mayor, the arena hosts professional lacrosse games and serves as the training facility of the Baltimore Blast, the city's indoor soccer team and frequent Major Indoor Soccer League champion.

● Canton Waterfront Park is a special place. While all the surrounding streets continue to be swept up in a tide of gentrification, here you can still grab a shady spot, feel the breezes off the water, and simply relax. A favorite haunt of couples, families, and city dwellers looking for some peace and quiet, the park offers a perfect place to check out the water views across the Patapsco (yes, that's Fort McHenry across the water) and watch the crabbers and fishermen pulling their catch from the murky waters off the Waterfront Promenade.

Be sure to check out the attractive Korean War Memorial at the north edge of the park, just off Boston St. Dedicated in 1990, the granite memorial, set into the ground, contains the names of the 527 Marylanders who died during the conflict, as well as the names of those still officially considered missing in action. The center of the memorial features a map of Korea, also in granite.

● Follow the Waterfront Promenade west, passing marinas and restaurants, including Bo Brooks, a great place for steamed crabs, until you come to Boston Street Pier Park. Enjoy this walk; while the city pulses to your right, looking left over the water forces you to slow down and take in the pleasing, lazy atmosphere. Plus, there's something really nice about hearing the lap of small waves in the middle of a city. You'll see much development along the water here; many of these condos and apartments are of newer construction, but some make use of older industrial buildings. The development began full bore in the 1980s, with developers recognizing the attractiveness and reclamation potential of waterside living along what had languished for many years as a rather unattractive swath of spent industrial sites. Today, the waterside development, far more tastefully done than otherwise, wraps around the entire water line all the way through Fells Point (Walk 6), Harbor East (Walk 5), and into the Inner Harbor (Walk 4).

● At Boston Street Pier Park, cross Boston St. at the American Can Company development (you'll see the Safeway across Boston). This is the site of what was in its time the largest can manufacturer in the United States. The American Can Company started in 1901, preceded here by the Norton Tin Can and Plate Company, whose main building still stands and dates from 1895 (one block west of the Safeway). Today, you'll find plenty of shops and restaurants, another success story in reclaiming old and once-contaminated industrial sites and reusing them to serve the needs and wants of city dwellers.

● Your first street off Boston, south and east of the Can Company complex, is O'Donnell St. Take it heading east, moving in the direction of St. Casimir's school and church. St. Casimir's dates to 1902 and was erected to serve Canton's growing Polish immigrant community. Go to the front of the church to see this beautiful limestone building's most impressive external features; take note of the two cupolas holding bell towers and carved with niches where

John O'Donnell, Canton's founder

Back Story

Few things scream Baltimore more than the one-eyed, mustachioed Mr. Boh, an icon since his introduction in 1936. Since its inception in 1885, National Bohemian has been proclaiming good tidings from "The Land of Pleasant Living." The brand came packing wacky and wonderful cartoon pitchmen beyond the famous one-eyed barkeep, including an oyster, a turtle, a seagull or duck (or blue bird) wearing a ship captain's hat, a pelican, and a vaguely colonial chap toting a banjo. All weirdness and all great fun. At one time, the brewery's president also owned the Baltimore Orioles and the two became intertwined, with Natty Boh on tap at all O's games. Yes, the O's on the radio, a pile of crabs, and a case of Natty Boh: the essential ingredients for Baltimore nirvana.

9-foot statues of St. Francis of Assisi and St. Anthony of Padua gaze down with benevolence. Inside, see the 14 stained glass windows, a series of impressive murals, and a main altar modeled on the one at the Basilica of St. Anthony in Padua, Italy.

● Moving east along O'Donnell St., you'll see where much of Canton's revitalization has taken place. You'll find an eclectic assortment of shops and restaurants, all spillover from the inland portion of the neighborhood's focal point, O'Donnell Square, which you will reach in one block. Once the site of Canton Market (1859), O'Donnell Square is where you'll find locals darting in and out of the shops and bars or simply taking a spot on one of the many benches in the shaded green space. (If there's a big soccer match taking place somewhere in the world, Claddagh's Pub, on the square, is the best place in the city to take it in.) In the middle of it all is the statue to the father of Canton, Captain John O'Donnell, who settled in Baltimore-Town in 1780 and initiated trade between Baltimore and Canton, China, in 1785, thus the name. Of course, the local stress here is on the first syllable, "CAN-ton," as opposed to the Chinese "Can-TON." Most of Canton was originally O'Donnell's waterside plantation. (It was on that plantation that local Betsy Patterson met Prince Jerome Bonaparte, Napoléon's brother, in 1803. They married two years later. Archbishop Carroll presided over the ceremony.) Look for the unique "keyhole" house on the north edge of the square, just before S. Ellwood Ave. This private home stands out for its beautiful stone construction and circular covered entranceway.

● After a respite in O'Donnell Square, continue heading east, toward the granite church on the east side of the square. This is the home of the Messiah English Lutheran Church, dating to 1890. Behind the church is the Canton branch of the Enoch Pratt Library. This branch, on the National Register of Historic Places, was one of the system's four original branches and has been in continuous use since 1886, making it the city's oldest branch. Its architect, Charles Carson, designed many Baltimore landmarks (including the Mount Vernon Methodist Church; see Walk 16) and was responsible for the keyhole house noted above. *Note:* the library is undergoing renovation slated to last until January 2014.

● Continue moving east on O'Donnell St., taking note of Canton's residential profile: tidy, two-story row homes of brick, stone, and the occasional Formstone (a type of cement designed to imitate stone). Be on the lookout also for painted screens (for the lowdown on painted screens and Formstone, both beloved institutions of Baltimore kitsch, see Walk 9: Patterson Park to Highlandtown). The houses here and on bordering blocks were built primarily in the late 19th and early 20th centuries for the large influx of blue-collar immigrant workers, mostly German, Greek, Irish, Polish, and Welsh. Later waves brought immigrants from farther east: Lithuanians, Russians, Ukrainians.

As you move east, you'll see one of the city's most iconic images, the illuminated one-eyed Mr. Boh (see "Back Story" on the previous page). Eight blocks from the library is S. Conkling St., where you'll find Natty Boh Tower, named for the adored local brew that has now been embraced by a younger generation of Baltimoreans both paying homage to the city's past and celebrating its present quirkiness and charm.

● You're now in the heart of Brewers Hill, an up-and-coming neighborhood that has seen some thoughtful and inventive reuse. This area is where National Brewery and Gunther Brewery operated for decades, beginning in the 1880s, churning out Gunther, Hamms, National Bohemian, National Premium, and Schaefer, among other brands. One of National's more popular outputs was Colt 45, named for Baltimore

Colts running back Jerry Hill, #45. It was here that the six-pack was invented, revolutionizing (cheap) beer consumption. Now, the old complex is used for retail, office, light industrial, and residential use, but reminders of its brewing past abound, with great nostalgia-inducing signage attached to the old brick buildings. To wander around the place, you can go one block north on S. Conkling, to Dillon St., and take a right. Here, breweriana abounds.

● Return to S. Conkling and head south, toward the harbor. Take the first right onto Elliott St., at the massive, brick Hamms Brewery building. Elliott St. reflects Canton's waterside roots, as the street was named for Jesse Duncan Elliott, the superintendent of the Philadelphia Navy Yard.

● Take your first left onto S. Baylis St. (Conkling and Baylis are the names of past leaders of the industrial Canton Company, as are street names Leakin and Gwynne). It was at the corner of O'Donnell and Baylis where George Pabst opened a small brewery in 1860. The next block south is Toone St., named in honor of a local saloon owner who in the early 1820s owned Toone's Pleasure Gardens, where patrons could grab a drink and watch the races at the nearby tracks.

Boston St. is the next block, and across Boston is Canton Crossing, where you began. If you're up for it, follow Clinton St. all the way south another quarter mile or so to its water end. A quarantine hospital used to stand here, as did a lighthouse. Visitors to Fort McHenry have no doubt noticed the Lehigh Cement Plant across the water; that is what stands at the end of Clinton St. now. Interestingly, so does the lighthouse, near the water's edge in front of the cement plant off Mertens Ave. What you can see there now isn't the original, however, which was constructed in 1831. Sadly, that lighthouse, Chesapeake's first electric lighthouse, was demolished in 1926 after it was deemed superfluous. What stands there now is a faithful reproduction, erected in the 1980s.

POINTS OF INTEREST (START TO FINISH)

Clarence "Du" Burns Arena 1301 S. Ellwood Ave., 443-573-2450

Canton Waterfront Park 2903 Boston St.

Korean War Memorial Canton Waterfront Park, 2903 Boston St.

Bo Brooks 2701/150 Lighthouse Point, 410-558-0202

American Can Company thecancompany.com, 2400 Boston St., 443-573-4460

St. Casimir's stcasimir.org, 2800 O'Donnell St., 410-276-1981

O'Donnell Square 2900 block of O'Donnell St.

Claddagh's Pub claddaghonline.com, 2918 O'Donnell St., 410-522-4220

Messiah English Lutheran Church messiahodsq.com, 1025 South Potomac St.,
410-324-4543

Enoch Pratt Free Library, Canton Branch prattlibrary.org/locations/canton,
1030 S. Ellwood Ave., 410-545-7130

Brewers Hill brewershill.net, Conkling St. to O'Donnell and Dillon Sts.

route summary

1. Start at Canton Crossing, S. Clinton St. south of Boston St.
2. Go north on S. Clinton and turn left onto Boston St.
3. Enter Canton Waterfront Park.
4. Head west on the Harbor Promenade.
5. Cross Boston St. north of Boston Street Pier Park.
6. Enter the American Can Company complex.
7. Go east on O'Donnell St.
8. Explore Brewers Hill at S. Conkling, O'Donnell, and Dillon Sts.
9. Go south on S. Conkling St.
10. Turn right onto Elliott St.
11. Turn left onto S. Baylis St.
12. Turn right onto Boston St.
13. Turn left onto S. Clinton St.

CONNECTING THE WALKS

From the American Can Company complex, Patterson Park (Walk 9) is five blocks due north. Once on the Harbor Promenade, stay on it heading west and you'll soon be in Fells Point (Walk 6).

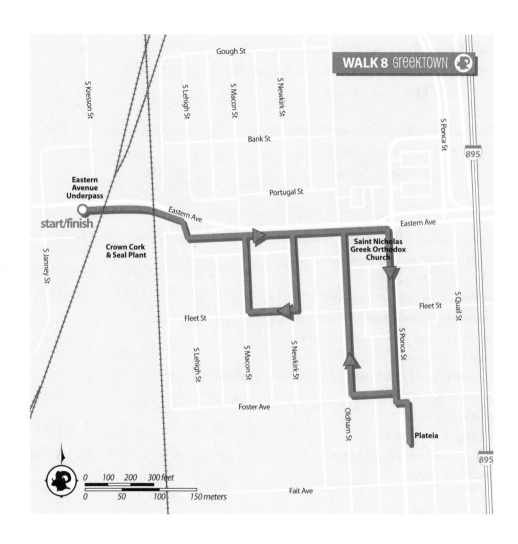

S Kresson St

Gough St

S Lehigh St

S Macon St

S Newkirk St

S Ponca St

895

Bank St

Eastern
Avenue
Underpass

Portugal St

Eastern Ave

Eastern Ave

start/finish

S Janney St

Crown Cork
& Seal Plant

Saint Nicholas
Greek Orthodox
Church

Fleet St

S Quail St

Fleet St

S Newkirk St

S Macon St

S Lehigh St

S Ponca St

Oldham St

Foster Ave

Plateia

0   100   200   300 feet

0   50   100   150 meters

Fait Ave

895

8 GreekTOWN: a LITTLe SLICe OF aTHeNS

BOUNDARIES: **Eastern Ave., S. Ponca St., Foster Ave.**
DISTANCE: **0.9 mile**
DIFFICULTY: **Easy**
PARKING: **Street parking all along route**
PUBLIC TRANSIT: **MTA bus #20 runs along Ponca St. MTA buses #s 10, 13, 22, and 30 run along Eastern Ave. (Future plans call for a red line extension of the Light Rail to run through Greektown.)**

Greektown, long known simply as The Hill (many old-timers still refer to their neighborhood this way), got its start in the 1890s. For many years, it was thought of primarily as a small eastern adjunct of neighboring Highlandtown. It has been called, variously, East Highlandtown, Highland Hills, and Bayview. Because a large influx of Greek immigrants settled here, in the 1980s the locals successfully petitioned the Baltimore City Council to officially change the name to Greektown. What's wonderful about Greektown today is that, unlike so many other ethnic enclaves where successive generations lit out for the suburbs, there is still an authentic Greek flavor here. This little neighborhood does not at all feel as if the Greeks are simply stopping in to manage their restaurants or attend church. So many of them still happily make their homes here. Yes, the neighborhood is changing a bit—you'll see several Latin restaurants now—but there are still Greeks galore. The result is that you can hear Greek being spoken from stoops, the food is authentic (and terrific), and the joyous outpourings you'll witness during the Greek Festival make this feel like a little slice of Athens in East Baltimore.

● Eastern Ave. is the main drag bisecting Greektown and the location for many of its favorite restaurants, so begin there, as close to the Eastern Avenue Underpass as possible. The mural on the underpass is worth checking out. It stretches one quarter of a mile and links Greektown with Highlandtown to the west, making it the largest mural in the city. The mural, which is on both sides of the street, depicts people engaged in activities typical of those living in these immigrant communities: Greek dancing, soccer, parades, bocce.

Back Story

It seems a somewhat simple thing, the bottle cap. Most of us think of them only as we're twisting or prying them off a beer bottle. But when Baltimore businessman William Painter invented a flanged metal cap in 1892, he revolutionized bottling. Now the world had a way to keep carbonated drinks fizzy. Crown Cork & Seal originally set up on Guilford Ave. (see Walk 21: Station North) but moved here to Greektown in 1904. When company president Charles E. McManus invented a cork lining for the bottle cap, the company took off and turned itself into the world's largest producer. A simple invention? Perhaps. But how many people, in Baltimore and around the world, have on a steamy summer day pried the cap off their favorite refreshing drink and listened with extreme satisfaction to the telltale hiss of freshness? Ahhhh.

● As you emerge from the underpass, where Lehigh St. intersects Eastern Ave., you'll see the first of many Greek flags to your right. Here, there are also American and Maryland flags; in some sections of Greektown, you'll see nothing but the blue and white of the Greek national flag and often a dozen or more grouped together. Behind these flags, also to your right and behind you a little, is the old hulk of an impressive industrial building. This was once the Crown Cork & Seal plant, which produced some 40 billion bottle caps a year and held the distinction of being the largest bottle cap factory in the world, employing upwards of 5,000 people. You can poke around the place today—though do so carefully. Large swaths of the complex look like they haven't been touched since the plant's closure in 1958. But other sections are now home to machine shops, coffee roasters, and woodworking shops. Also, perhaps fittingly, Bawlmer Craft Beers LLC has installed a brewery here.

● Return to Eastern Ave. and head east. You may as well follow the parade route used during Greek Independence Day celebrations every year at the end of March. The parade actually begins on the west side of the underpass, coming up Haven St. and following Eastern Ave. through the underpass. The parade is something to see: traditional dress, dancing, and music fill the air. And, of course, there's plenty of delicious food to sample.

- As you make your way up Eastern Ave., you'll immediately notice the profusion of Greek flags and restaurants. In this short stretch of Eastern, plus quick detours up side streets, you'll find no fewer than seven Greek restaurants, including the award-winning Acropolis; Zagat-rated and nationally known Samos; and a local favorite, Ikaros.

- When you reach Ponca St., take a right. At the end of the block, you'll come to the Saint Nicholas Greek Orthodox Church. This is in many ways the neighborhood's central meeting point, and not only on worship days. The church was founded in 1953 and has grown to accommodate more than a thousand parishioners. Services are still held largely in ancient Greek. The church sponsors the annual Greek Folk Festival in June, four days focusing on Hellenic culture. More than 30 years strong, it is not only one of the Mid-Atlantic's longest-running celebrations of Greek culture, it's also one of the biggest, drawing visitors from all over the region.

- Continue another one and a half blocks south on S. Ponca St. to the 700 block. On the left, just past Foster Ave., is the Plateia. This is the building where locals show-case Greek-related and Greektown-inspired artistic performances: concerts, foreign films, plays, readings.

- Return to Foster Ave. and take a left. Greektown is a low-crime and close-knit area, encompassing both the southeastern city police district and Johns Hopkins Bayview Medical Center. Proximity to major highways—I-895 runs through and I-95 forms the eastern border of the neighborhood—also makes it ripe for renewed investment. To that end, a new town home development is in the works (as of 2012, construction had just begun) just one block west.

- At the next block, Oldham St., take a right. Midway up the block, you'll find a great Greek-themed mural to the right. Continue back to Eastern Ave. and take a left.

- The rest of the walk provides an opportunity to take in the more residential feel of Greektown. As you make your way down the main and side streets, you'll notice how tidy Greektown feels. Bowfront row houses with marble stoops where folks sit and chat—in Greek, in English, in Spanish—it's quintessential Baltimore. To take in just two of these residential blocks, take a left onto S. Newkirk St. from Eastern. Follow it one block to Fleet St. and take a right. Then take a right at the next block, S. Macon St., and follow it back to Eastern Ave. You will be just one and a half blocks from the Eastern Avenue Underpass.

POINTS OF INTEREST (START TO FINISH)

Eastern Avenue Underpass Between S. Haven St. and S. Lehigh St.

Crown Cork & Seal Plant Eastern Ave.

Acropolis acropolisbaltimore.com, 4718 Eastern Ave., 410-675-3384

Samos samosrestaurant.com, 600 Oldham St., 410-675-5292

Ikaros ikarosrestaurant.com, 4901 Eastern Ave., 410-633-3750

Saint Nicholas Greek Orthodox Church 520 S. Ponca St., 410-633-5020

Plateia 700 block of S. Ponca St.

ROUTE SUMMARY

1. Start at the Eastern Avenue Underpass.
2. Head east on Eastern Ave.
3. Turn right onto S. Ponca St.
4. Turn left onto Foster Ave.
5. Turn right onto Oldham St.
6. Turn left onto Eastern Ave.
7. Turn left onto S. Newkirk St.
8. Turn right onto Fleet St.
9. Turn right onto S. Macon St.
10. Turn left onto Eastern Ave.

CONNECTING THE WALKS

On the west side of the Eastern Avenue Underpass sits Highlandtown. It's five blocks to the Enoch Pratt Free Library's Southeast Anchor branch, where Walk 9: Patterson Park to Highlandtown intersects.

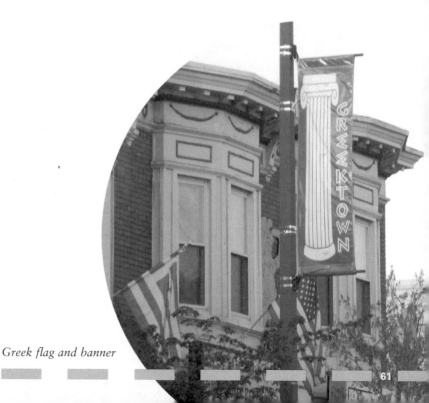

Greek flag and banner

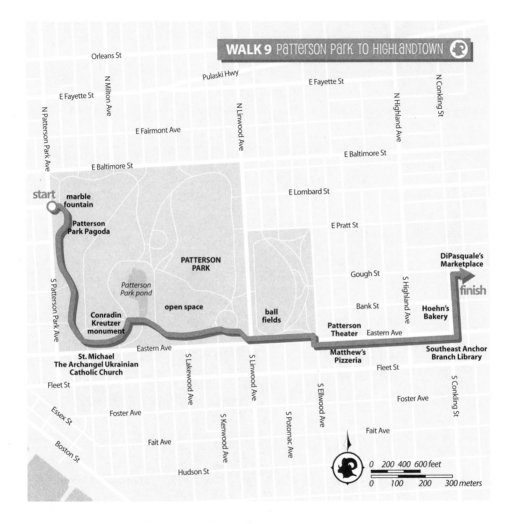

WALK 9 Patterson Park to Highlandtown

Orleans St

Pulaski Hwy

E Fayette St

N Conkling St

N Highland Ave

E Fayette St

N Milton Ave

N Patterson Park Ave

E Fairmont Ave

N Linwood Ave

E Baltimore St

E Baltimore St

E Lombard St

start   marble
         fountain

Patterson
Park Pagoda

E Pratt St

DiPasquale's
Marketplace

PATTERSON
PARK

Gough St

finish

S Patterson Park Ave

Patterson
Park pond

open space

ball
fields

Bank St

S Highland Ave

Hoehn's
Bakery

Conradin
Kreutzer
monument

Eastern Ave

Patterson
Theater

Eastern Ave

St. Michael
The Archangel Ukrainian
Catholic Church

S Lakewood Ave

S Linwood Ave

Matthew's
Pizzeria

Southeast Anchor
Branch Library

Fleet St

Fleet St

S Ellwood Ave

Foster Ave

Essex St

Foster Ave

S Kenwood Ave

S Potomac Ave

Fait Ave

S Conkling St

Boston St

Fait Ave

Hudson St

0   200 400 600 feet

0   100   200   300 meters

9 PATTERSON PARK TO HIGHLANDTOWN: FROM BALTIMORE'S BACKYARD TO VILNIUS, LITHUANIA

BOUNDARIES: S. Patterson Park Ave., Eastern Ave., S. Conkling St., Gough St.
DISTANCE: 2.3 miles
DIFFICULTY: Moderate
PARKING: Parking all along route, with some residential restrictions. Travel one or two streets off the main thoroughfares (such as Eastern Ave.) for free parking.
PUBLIC TRANSIT: MTA bus #7 runs north–south along S. Patterson Park Ave.; MTA buses #10 and #30 run east–west along Eastern Ave.; MTA buses #s 10, 13, and 22 stop at S. Conkling St. and Eastern Ave. at the Enoch Pratt Free Library's Southeast Anchor branch.

Patterson Park is an urban oasis of 137 acres and is known as "Baltimore's Best Backyard." Its birth as a park almost 200 years ago (1827) was already a little late in coming: the earliest colonial residents had begun setting down roots there in 1669. And in between, it served an integral role in the defense of the nation. During the War of 1812, as the British were burning the Capitol and bombarding Fort McHenry, some 20,000 troops and 100 cannons arrayed on Patterson Park's Hampstead Hill repelled advancing British soldiers who took one look at the impressive martial display and retreated to their ships in the harbor, thus halting further inland incursions. Even after its founding as a park, Patterson Park served as a fortification yet again, during the Civil War. After more tough times in the 1980s and early 1990s—earning a reputation as a center of drug activity—Patterson Park has blossomed once again into the true recreation center it was designed to be in the early 19th century. Today, it's all swimming, fishing, soccer, festivals, dog walkers, baby strollers, and myriad ethnicities enjoying this promised green space. This walk begins in Patterson Park and takes in neighboring Highlandtown, a neighborhood that has always been—and continues to be—a first stop for waves of immigrants to the United States. Plus, it has Frank Zappa; more on that later.

● **Begin where E. Lombard St. ends at S. Patterson Park Ave. and enter the park; you'll see four decorative stone pillars and a pathway there. The credit for Patterson Park's renaissance belongs primarily to the Friends of Patterson Park, a nonprofit formed in 1998 "to promote, protect and advocate for our treasured common ground so that it** can be enjoyed for generations to come." The organization's white brick headquarters is just to the left of the entrance. Pop in and see what activities are planned.

Straight ahead you'll see the marble fountain, the park's first architectural element, designed in 1865 by George Frederick, who also designed Baltimore's grand City Hall. The fountain plays host to Patterson Park's annual wine-tasting event.

● Head to the right of the fountain and behold the four-story octagonal Patterson Park Pagoda, a true architectural gem. Superintendent of Parks Charles Latrobe designed the structure, which was originally known as the Observation Tower, in 1890. This striking hybrid of Oriental and Victorian design, graced by beautiful stained glass, sits on Hampstead Hill and provides scenic views of downtown and the harbor. These views help explain the line of cannons, marked 1814, in front of the pagoda. These cannons delineate the chain of fortifications that once ran from the harbor all the way to present day Johns Hopkins Hospital and helped repel the British. The cannon directly in front of the pagoda, erected in 1914, marks the centennial commemoration of its original placement and stands as a memorial to Commodore John Rodgers, commander of the ground troops stationed on Hampstead Hill. Next to this cannon stands a bronze statue of two small children, also erected in 1914, commemorating the centennial of the writing of "The Star-Spangled Banner." The Pagoda is open for tours 12–6 p.m. on Sundays between April and October and hosts free summer concerts. The view over the city from the top is something to behold.

● There are dozens of pathways through the park, so take them at your leisure, but a recommended route from the pagoda will take you south toward Eastern Ave., where, just three blocks east of S. Patterson Park Ave., you'll see the beautiful gold-colored onion domes of St. Michael The Archangel Ukrainian Catholic Church, modeled after a similar church in Kiev. It's a nice little slice of Eastern Europe in Baltimore. Continuing eastward within the park, you'll pass the monument to 19th-century German composer Conradin Kreutzer. The United Singers of Baltimore won the bust in 1915 in Saengerfest, a German cultural competition. This route will also take you to the southern edge of the Patterson Park pond. This is a catch-and-release pond (requiring a fishing license) created in 1864 after the removal of military emplacements. You can walk across the pond on a wooden boardwalk. No doubt you'll see ducks congregating here. But ducks are just a small part of the vigorous avian life in Patterson

Park. More than 50 bird species, and another 100 varieties, have been spotted, mostly members of the thrush, warbler, and sparrow families. But there have also been many birds spotted only rarely in the area, such as the gadwall, blue-winged teal, American bittern, dark-eyed junco, and merlin. (Visit pattersonpark.com and baltimorebirdclub.org for more information on birding at Patterson Park.) Three bird species mate and breed here: red-winged blackbirds, mallards, and wood ducks. You can join a bird walk the last Saturday of every month at 8 a.m., sponsored by the Audubon Society's Maryland/D.C. chapter.

- As you head through the park, you'll be passing a good number of mature trees. This is no happy accident. As early as 1835, Revolutionary War participant William Patterson (the man who lends his name to the park) was planting some 200 trees on his original 6 acres of parkland. (Odd note: one of his daughters, Betsy, married Napoléon Bonaparte's brother—you can't make this stuff up.) Today, there are more than 1,500 trees in Patterson Park. The majority are linden, maple, and oak, but there are more than 50 species. The result is a wonderfully colorful show in spring and fall.

- Continuing eastward, you'll come to the large open space that every June for the past 30 years has hosted Latinofest, the city's largest celebration of all things Latin: food, dance, art, music. It's a wonderful event. To the north, you'll pass the Patterson Park pool as well as the Dominic "Mimi" DiPietro Family Skating Center. Still close to Eastern Ave., just before S. Linwood Ave., check out the imposing 1951 monument to Polish soldier and patriot Kazimierz (Casimir) Pulaski, who, after spending his early years fighting the Russians, was exiled and wound up fighting for the fledgling American nation in the Revolutionary

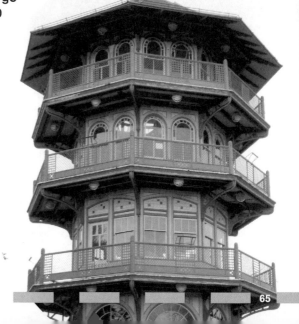

Patterson Park Pagoda

Back Story

The story of the Frank Zappa bust's journey to this corner of Baltimore is a rather odd one, befitting the strange but talented musician. It begins on a faraway city street corner in Vilnius, Lithuania. After Lithuania's break from the Soviet Union, the citizenry began systematically dismantling the many busts of Lenin, Marx, and other Soviet figures that dotted the city. In one such neighborhood, Uzupis, a local civil servant founded the Frank Zappa Fan Club and commissioned a sculptor who used to make a trade in busts of Stalin to do one of Zappa. President Vaclav Havel presided over the dedication, where a

military brass band belted out renditions of Zappa songs. Weird? Yes. Perfect for the strangeness of Baltimore? Absolutely. And so, after Zappa's popularity grew tremendously in Lithuania, the Lithuanian nonprofit organization ZAPPART offered a replica of that bust to the city of Zappa's birth in 2008. The mayor of Vilnius at the time signed on, writing, "I hope that replication of the original statue of Frank Zappa in Vilnius and bringing it to Baltimore will perpetuate the memory of one of the greatest artists of the century." And there you have it.

War. He earned a place of valor on the battlefields of America, once saving George Washington's life at Brandywine, and came to be known as the Father of the American Cavalry. This beautiful monument depicts Pulaski as he led his cavalry force during the Battle of Savannah.

- Cross S. Linwood Ave., passing baseball diamonds to your left, and link up with the main commercial strip in the area, Eastern Ave., just after S. Ellwood Ave.

- For the next six blocks, be on the lookout for many shopping and eating opportunities (but if you like Italian, hold off on eating until the end of this walk). Matthew's Pizzeria, a city favorite since 1943 (often voted Best Pizza in the City) is just up ahead to the right, at 3131 Eastern Ave. Across the street is the historic Patterson Movie Theater; look for the vertical Art Deco marquee. The theater is home today to the Creative Alliance (CA). Founded in 1995 as the Fells Point Creative Alliance, this nonprofit focuses on nurturing and showcasing the arts as a necessary part of the fabric of daily life. After the CA began to expand rapidly, it needed a new, large space. The theater, built in 1930, was the perfect spot. The CA moved there in 2003 and has established two art galleries, a 180-seat theater, a classroom, and a media lab. Coolest of all (and pretty unique) is that the CA also houses eight live-in artists who apply and are awarded studio and living space for terms of one to three years for a more than reasonable monthly rent.

● Continue eastward along Eastern Ave. You're in the heart of Highlandtown, a once and still thriving immigrant neighborhood. Where it used to be the draw for Europeans—Germans, Poles, Ukrainians—today it attracts primarily Latin Americans and Africans. Though not as Latinized as Upper Fells Point (see Walk 6: Fells Point), the area's Latin influence extends beyond Patterson Park's Latinofest; you'll notice many Spanish-language signs up and down Eastern Ave., as well as Latin-themed mercados and stores selling Latin music and soccer gear.

● Continue a few more blocks until you reach S. Conkling St. On the right is the Southeast Anchor branch of the Enoch Pratt Free Library. Opened in 2007, it was the system's first new library in 30 years. Today, it serves—as all libraries do—as a great neighborhood hub. In front of the library, on the corner of Eastern Ave. and S. Conkling St., is one of the city's newer monuments, and it's one that strikes a lot of unsuspecting visitors as a bit odd: on top of a 12-foot pole sits the bronzed head of Frank Zappa with his trademark long mustache and longer ponytail. The genre-bending and incredibly prolific musician is justly remembered not only for his music but also for his vigorous 1985 defense of First Amendment rights before a Senate subcommittee considering music censorship. He produced and recorded some 60 albums either as a solo artist or with his band, The Mothers of Invention, during a career that lasted more than 30 years. On August 9, 2007, then-Mayor Sheila Dixon proclaimed that date "Frank Zappa Day" in Baltimore in part because "The City of Baltimore is proud of its rich musical heritage, and is honored to claim the prolific composer, musician, author, and film director Frank Zappa as a native of our fair city. . . ." Zappa was born in Baltimore in 1940 and is one of a long number of musical greats to come out of Charm City. The pages of this book make note of many Baltimore artists and musicians, but Zappa stands out because of the uniqueness of his vision. His music was so completely distinctive that its influence spans an incredible spectrum of musicians working today. He was inducted into the Rock and Roll Hall of Fame in 1995, two years after his death. The text of that induction reads, in part: "Frank Zappa was rock and roll's sharpest musical mind and most astute social critic. He was the most prolific composer of his age, and he bridged genres—rock, jazz, classical, avant-garde and even novelty music—with masterful ease." For the kooky story on how the bust of Zappa came to be here, see "Back Story" on page 66.

- Cross Eastern Ave. from the library, heading north on S. Conkling St. Walk two blocks to Gough St. (pronounced "Goff" and named for Harry Gough, a wealthy Marylander and owner of the Perry Hall plantation in the late 1700s) and take a right. Just up the street on the left, at 3700 Gough St., is DiPasquale's Marketplace, an exquisite Italian market, in operation since 1914. While Baltimore's Little Italy gets understandable and deserved recognition as the place to go for terrific Italian food, this out-of-the-way market is a real find—the sort of place in-the-know Baltimoreans go for a wonderful and mouthwatering array of Italian food.

- To return to your starting point at Patterson Park, you can take Gough St. west or go one block south to Bank St. and take that west. Be sure to stop off at Hoehn's Bakery, on the corner of Bank and Conkling, for some phenomenal baked goods. Here since 1927, the owners have used the same massive brick hearth oven originally installed by German immigrant William Hoehn, who started the business. MTA buses run along both Gough and Bank, but it's only 10 short blocks back to the park's western end. Either of these streets will give you view to another Baltimore oddity: the lingering attachment to what that lover of kitsch and purveyor of weird, director John Waters, called "the polyester of brick": Formstone. Introduced in Baltimore in 1937, Formstone is a type of cement applied to house exteriors, such as those made of brick, and then sculpted to resemble stone (yes, people slathered over their brick in favor of something not nearly as attractive). Waters coproduced the documentary on Formstone, *Little Castles.* Of course, it has been so maligned and so consistently dismissed as hopelessly uncool that now Formstone has become, perhaps inevitably, something that newer and younger (mostly hipster) homeowners are proud to sport. If you're lucky enough to catch a Formstone house that also boasts a painted screen, you are in Baltimore kitsch nirvana.

Another Baltimore tradition, the painted screen, began when Czech immigrant William Oktavec painted a wire screen in 1913. It immediately caught on: the pastoral scene on the outside, still allowing breezes to pass through (the trick and the art is to paint on the wires, not plug up the holes), effectively prevented anyone from seeing in. Soon enough, virtually every Baltimore row home in the area (Highlandtown, Canton, Little Bohemia, Fells Point) sported a painted screen—what better way to distinguish your home from the abundant copycat row houses up and down Baltimore's residential streets? While virtually all of those original screens have disappeared, many torn down as hopeless nods to the inglorious past, they have regained currency in recent years, with many Baltimoreans paying good money to resurrect them—as a paean to that glorious past.

POINTS OF INTEREST (START TO FINISH)

Patterson Park Pagoda (Friends of Patterson Park) pattersonpark.com, 27 S. Patterson Park Ave., 410-276-3676

Matthew's Pizzeria matthewspizza.com, 3131 Eastern Ave., 410-276-8755

Creative Alliance creativealliance.org, 3134 Eastern Ave., 410-276-1651

Southeast Anchor Library (and Frank Zappa shrine) 3601 Eastern Ave., 410-396-1580

DiPasquale's Marketplace dipasquales.com, 3700 Gough St., 410-276-6787

Hoehn's Bakery hoehnsbakery.com, 400 S. Conkling St., 410-675-2884

ROUTE SUMMARY

1. Start at Patterson Park (at the E. Lombard St. and S. Patterson Park Ave. entrance).
2. Move southeastward through Patterson Park.
3. Cross S. Ellwood Ave. and join Eastern Ave.
4. Walk six blocks to S. Conkling St. to the Southeast Branch of the Enoch Pratt.
5. Take S. Conkling St. two blocks north to a right on Gough St.
6. Take either Gough St. or Bank St. west about 10 blocks to return to Patterson Park.

St. Michael The Archangel Ukrainian Catholic Church

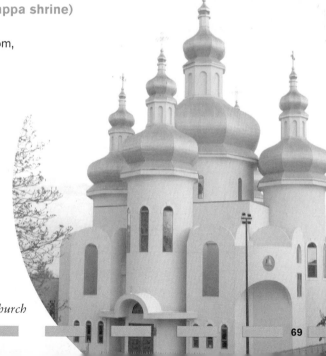

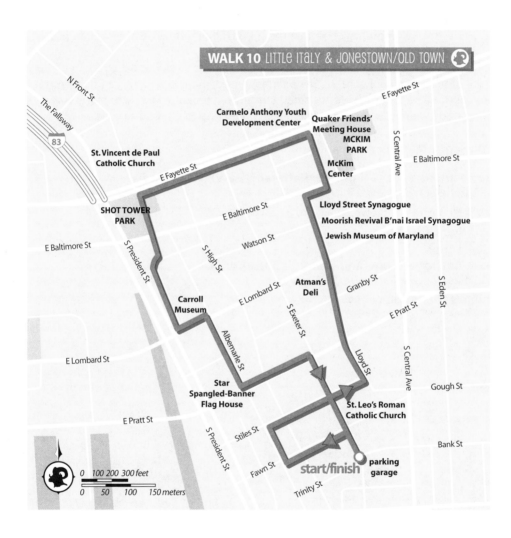

N Front St

The Fallsway

83

St. Vincent de Paul
Catholic Church

E Fayette St

E Fayette St

Carmelo Anthony Youth
Development Center

Quaker Friends'
Meeting House
MCKIM
PARK

McKim
Center

S Central Ave

E Fayette St

E Baltimore St

SHOT TOWER
PARK

E Baltimore St

Watson St

E Baltimore St

E Baltimore St

S President St

S High St

Lloyd Street Synagogue

Moorish Revival B'nai Israel Synagogue

Jewish Museum of Maryland

Carroll
Museum

E Lombard St

Atman's
Deli

Granby St

S Eden St

S Exeter St

E Pratt St

E Lombard St

Albemarle St

Lloyd St

S Central Ave

Gough St

Star
Spangled-Banner
Flag House

St. Leo's Roman
Catholic Church

E Pratt St

Stiles St

Bank St

S President St

Fawn St

start/finish

parking
garage

Trinity St

0 100 200 300 feet

0   50   100 150 meters

10 LITTLE ITALY & JONESTOWN/OLD TOWN: WHERE IT ALL BEGAN

BOUNDARIES: **E. Fayette St., Aisquith St., Lloyd St., S. Exeter St., Fawn St., N. Front St.**
DISTANCE: **1.3 miles**
DIFFICULTY: **Moderate**
PARKING: **Street parking along route and public garages in Little Italy (S. Exeter St. and Bank St. and E. Pratt St. before Albemarle St.)**
PUBLIC TRANSIT: **MTA bus #11 stops at Fawn St. and President St.; MTA buses #s 7, 10, and 30 run east–west along Pratt St.; the Charm City Circulator Orange runs throughout Old Town and the Green runs through Little Italy; the Shot Tower Metro stop is between President St. and S. Front St.**

Jonestown is in some respects where Baltimore began. The Englishman David Jones built his house on the banks of a stream that would later take his name, the Jones Falls, in 1661. Jones's house rested on the east side of the falls. By 1729, the surrounding area was bustling and local inhabitants lobbied the colonial legislature for a charter. The wealthy Carrolls donated 60 acres, and Baltimore City received its charter in 1729, named for Cecil Calvert, the 2nd Lord Baltimore and the founder of the Colony of Maryland. The earliest city planners began laying out Baltimore on the west side of Jones's waterway. By 1732, they began laying out the streets in Jonestown, on the east side. A bridge along Gay Street linked the two, and Jonestown then became known as Old Town. Though certainly quite different in appearance today, Jonestown still exists and the neighborhood still contains some of Baltimore's oldest man-made structures. This walk has plenty of historical riches, with no fewer than eight sites listed on the National Register of Historic Places. But before all that history, take a walk around the gustatory and olfactory enchantment of adjacent Little Italy, long home to one of the best collections of culinary delights anywhere on the East Coast.

Note: the small section of this walk that takes in the McKim School and the Friends' Meeting House sits on a somewhat neglected edge of town; some people might be a bit uncomfortable strolling here. That said, I have never had any troubles in the area.

● Begin on S. Exeter St. and Bank St. There is plenty of parking—both garage and street—here. Down Bank St. you'll see the 1866 Canal Street Malthouse, a mid-19th-century malt warehouse for what was once a collection of nearby breweries, today converted to upscale condos. Continue north on S. Exeter St., passing the tidy brick and Formstone row homes of Little Italy. The neighborhood got its ethnic flavor from a wave of Genoese immigrants in the 1850s. Many people know this neighborhood as a premier destination for food—you'll have your choice of almost 30 restaurants—but some folks tend to forget that this is a residential neighborhood too. There's a terrific website for Little Italy, littleitalymd.com, where you can find tons of information on restaurants, a walking map, an explanation of bocce, and anecdotal reminiscences from people who grew up in the neighborhood.

● At the next block, take a left onto Fawn St. The street was named to commemorate the cartel ship *Fawn,* which saw action in the War of 1812. As you head toward the harbor on Fawn St., you'll begin to pass the ubiquitous Italian restaurants. Many have been here for generations and earned reputations as wonderful eateries. With so many choices so close together (many of them literally sharing walls), if a restaurant fails to deliver, it won't be around for long. The result is consistently high-quality dining, year after year. Everybody has a favorite, and it's beyond my capacity to say which is the best. (That said, my wife could eat Ciao Bella's Shrimp Ricardo every day of the week.)

● The business end of Little Italy is fairly compact, so take time to check out the menus at the establishments on all the intersecting streets. But to continue this walk, stay on Fawn St., passing High St., and take a right onto Albemarle St. The street probably got its name from George Monck, the Duke of Albermarle, who was the English general primarily responsible for elevating Charles II to the British throne in the 17th century. But the street has a little hometown aristocracy attached to it as well: just as you turned onto Albemarle St., on the right at #245 is the house where Baltimore Mayor Thomas J. D'Alesandro Jr. was born and lived his whole life. The son of Italian immigrants, D'Alesandro served in Congress from 1939 to 1947 and served as Charm City's mayor from 1947 to 1959. His son Thomas J. D'Alesandro III followed him as mayor, serving from 1967 to 1971. But it was D'Alesandro III's little sister whose name rings the most bells; she's Nancy Pelosi, the country's first female Speaker of the House. She, too, grew up at 245 Albemarle St. Many of the neighborhood old-timers still remember "Little Nancy" from when she was just a kid running the streets. She's honored with a street sign declaring this portion of Albemarle St. "Via Nancy D'Alesandro Pelosi."

- An antique brick tower looms ahead; you'll be there on your return route. For now, take the next right, onto Stiles St., named for Captain George Stiles, a War of 1812 veteran and later Baltimore mayor. This first block, at High St. and Stiles St., is where you can catch open-air movies every Friday evening in July and August, including everyone's favorite, the classic *Cinema Paradiso*. You'll pass a bocce court to the left, and if you're lucky a game will be in full swing. If so, you'll swear you're in the Old Country.

- Continue on Stiles St., passing S. Exeter St., and you'll see the neighborhood's holy linchpin on the right, St. Leo's Roman Catholic Church. The church began in 1881 and is listed as a National Historic Shrine. The church used to run the St. Leo School, but it closed in 1980 after almost 100 years.

- Pass St. Leo's and continue to the next block, Lloyd St., and take a left. You're now leaving Little Italy and skirting the edge of historic Old Town, home to some of Baltimore's earliest structures. Continue on Lloyd St., passing E. Pratt St. Baltimoreans familiar with the area will remember when this part of town was an eyesore. But new housing in these blocks has really spruced up the area. Continue on Lloyd St. to E. Lombard St. (If for some reason, you didn't fill up in Little Italy, the famous Atman's Deli is on the left, at 1019 E. Lombard. An institution for almost 100 years, Atman's has earned a reputation as the best of the best along Baltimore's famed Corned Beef Row. Just a couple of blocks west, on Lombard St., somewhere near High St., Edgar Allan Poe was discovered in October 1849, fevered and delirious. He would die soon after being transported to nearby Church Hospital.

- Staying on Lloyd St., but crossing E. Lombard St., you'll see on the right

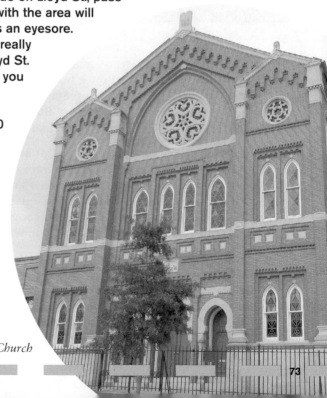

St. Leo's Roman Catholic Church

Back Story

Charles Carroll lends his name to many Maryland places: Carroll County, Carrollton, New Carrollton, and more. But he doesn't enjoy a great national reputation, which is a shame. He was a fascinating man whose influence on early America can't be overstated. Born in Annapolis in 1737, he publicly sparred with the Governor, who had usurped the Maryland General Assembly in 1772. His popularity for this act led to his election as Maryland's representative at the Continental Congress. He then helped to draft the constitution of Maryland and became the country's first elected Catholic senator, serving until 1792. All of this would have been enough to fill the life of any early American. But Carroll lived for another 40 years—serving as a director of the B&O Railroad and helping to establish the C&O Canal, the First and Second National Banks, Georgetown University in Washington, and many other public and private projects. When he died in 1832, he was 95 years old, a long veteran of the American Revolution who had lived a simply extraordinary life.

three important and historic buildings in succession. First is the redbrick Moorish Revival B'nai Israel Synagogue, built in 1876 by the Orthodox German-Jewish congregation Chizuk Amuno. The congregation sold the building in 1895 to the B'nai Israel congregation, made up primarily of Russian immigrants. It still functions today, making it the state's oldest continuous-use Orthodox synagogue.

Arches to the left connect it to another brick building, the more modern Jewish Museum of Maryland. The museum boasts the country's largest collection of regional Jewish Americana, focusing on centuries of Jewish life in Baltimore, the state of Maryland, and the United States. The museum has been in operation for 50 years, but perhaps its greatest historical function is as the overseer of the Lloyd Street Synagogue, just a few feet away across Watson St.

The Greek Revival–style Lloyd Street Synagogue was designed by Baltimore architect Robert Cary Long Jr. and built in 1845 by the Baltimore Hebrew Congregation. It was Maryland's first synagogue and is the nation's third oldest. The Baltimore Hebrew Congregation occupied the building until 1889, when it became St. John the Baptist Roman Catholic Church. This arrangement lasted until 1905; then the Orthodox Lithuanian Shomrei Mishmeres HaKodesh used the building until 1963. Today, the

Jewish Museum offers tours of both the Lloyd Street Synagogue and the B'nai Israel Synagogue every Sunday, Tuesday, Wednesday, and Thursday at 1 and 2:30 p.m.

● When you've checked out the synagogues and museum, follow Lloyd St. a few more feet to where it dead-ends at E. Baltimore St. and take a right. A hundred yards or so ahead on the left is McKim Park, anchored on Aisquith St. by the McKim Center. This striking building looks like it would be more at home in Athens, and there's a reason for that: its design was inspired by both the Propylaea, which was the monumental gateway to the Acropolis, and the Temple of Hephaestus, a Doric temple still standing in the Agora of Athens. This building was the original home of the McKim Free School, begun in 1821 (the building you see here was erected in 1833). It was Baltimore's first free school, and one of the first in the country as well. The building was designed by Baltimore architects William Howard and William Small, and according to the center's website, mckimcenter .org, it has been called "the most perfect example of Doric architecture in the U.S." The school served primarily immigrant children and remained in use almost until the 20th century, when its purpose was subsumed by the city's free public education system.

● Walk behind the McKim Center down Aisquith St. The street is one of the older ones in the city, named in the first years of the 1800s, probably for William Aisquith, the father of Ned Aisquith, assassin of a British general at the battle of North Point in 1814. To the right, just before you hit the major thoroughfare of E. Fayette St., you'll see a building even older than the McKim Center; this humble brick structure is the Quaker Friends' Meeting House. It remains the city's oldest religious-use structure, dating to 1781. The great city patron Johns Hopkins worshipped here, as did the B&O's first president, Philip E. Thomas.

● Take a left onto E. Fayette St. On the first block to the right, across the median, is the Carmelo Anthony Youth Development Center. Baltimore native and National Basketball Association all-star Carmelo Anthony donated $1.5 million for its creation; it serves the disadvantaged youth of East Baltimore.

● Continue west on E. Fayette St. for four blocks to the can't-miss Phoenix Shot Tower. This building is truly a national treasure; indeed, it's one of only three like it in the country. It stands 234 feet tall and is made up of more than a million bricks. When it was built in 1828, it was the country's tallest building. Its function was to create drop shot for smaller firearms and molded shot for larger weapons, such as cannons. Workers dropped molten lead from the top of the building through a long sieve and into a vat of cold water, creating the shape needed for the weaponry as it spun and cooled. The tower produced some 2.5 million pounds of shot annually. It remained in use until 1892. Tours of the tower are given every Saturday and Sunday at 4 p.m., leaving from the Carroll Mansion (see below).

Across E. Fayette St., you can see the Palladian bell tower of St. Vincent de Paul Catholic Church, the city's oldest continuous-use parish church, built in 1840.

● With the Shot Tower on your left, walk south along N. Front St. through Shot Tower Park. Cross E. Baltimore St. (N. Front St. becomes S. Front St. here). On the left, at 29 S. Front, is the gorgeous red iron façade of the building that used to house the City Life Museums, now sadly defunct. It's a private building now, rented out for weddings. But its 1840s cobblestone plaza is still a wonderful place to stroll. One museum that is still open, fortunately, is the Carroll Museum, just up to the left, at 800 E. Lombard St.

This building was the winter home of Charles Carroll, who would wind up as the country's last living (and only Catholic) signer of the Declaration of Independence. (For Carroll's biography, see "Back Story" on page 74.) The first house on this site was constructed between 1804 and 1808. Richard Caton, Charles Carroll's son-in-law, purchased it in 1820 after many additions to the original structure. Carroll himself spent many of his winters there, leaving his primary residence in Annapolis. After Carroll's and then the Catons' deaths in the mid-1800s, the house became a saloon and then a tenement apartment. For a decade in the early 1900s, the mansion functioned as a vocational school and ultimately became a recreation center in 1935. Today, Carroll Museums Inc. oversees the mansion and continues work on its restoration.

● Continue west on E. Lombard St. for another half block and take the first right onto Albemarle St. Go two blocks to E. Pratt St. and take a right. On your right is the Star-Spangled Banner Flag House, built in 1793. This unique museum concentrates on the story of the flag that inspired our national anthem and shines a light on Mary Pickersgill, the seamstress responsible for that star-spangled banner. As you pass through the museum, you'll see what life was like in early 19th-century Baltimore. It's a terrific children's museum. Although the original flag is at the Smithsonian in Washington, D.C., there is a fragment on display here.

● The point where you started is two blocks west on E. Pratt St. and three blocks south on S. Exeter St. Any southwestern route through Little Italy will get you there.

POINTS OF INTEREST (START TO FINISH)

St. Leo's Roman Catholic Church stleothegreatrcc.org, 227 S. Exeter St., 410-675-7275

Atman's Deli 1019 E. Lombard St.

B'nai Israel Synagogue bnaiisraelcongregation.org, 27 Lloyd St., 410-732-5454

The Jewish Museum of Maryland jhsm.org, 15 Lloyd St., 410-732-6400

The McKim School 1120 E. Baltimore St.

Old Town Friends' Meeting House 1201 E. Fayette St.

Phoenix Shot Tower 801 E. Fayette St., 410-837-5424

St. Vincent de Paul Catholic Church stvchurch.org, 120 N. Front St., 410-962-5078

Carroll Mansion carrollmuseums.org, 800 E. Lombard St., 410-605-2964

Star-Spangled Banner Flag House flaghouse.org, 844 E. Pratt St., 410-837-1793

ROUTE SUMMARY

1. Start at S. Exeter St. and Bank St.
2. Go north on S. Exeter St.
3. Turn left onto Fawn St.
4. Turn right onto Albemarle St.
5. Turn right onto Stiles St.
6. Turn left onto Lloyd St.
7. Turn right onto E. Baltimore St.
8. Turn left onto Aisquith St.
9. Turn left onto E. Fayette St.
10. Turn left onto N. Front St.
11. Turn left onto E. Lombard St.
12. Turn right onto Albemarle St.
13. Turn right onto E. Pratt St.

CONNECTING THE WALKS

Harbor East (Walk 5) begins just southeast of the starting point to this walk, at S. Caroline St. and Lancaster St. The Harbor East walk takes in the Reginald F. Lewis Museum of Maryland African American History and Culture, which shares the block of E. Pratt and Granby Street with the Star-Spangled Banner Flag House.

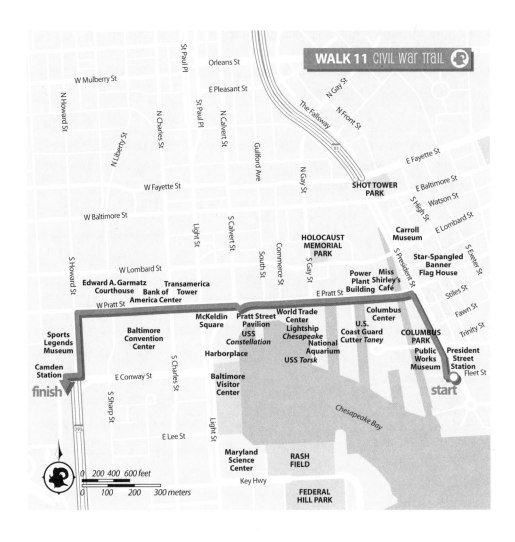

Orleans St

W Mulberry St

E Pleasant St

St Paul Pl

N Gay St

N Front St

The Fallsway

E Fayette St

N Howard St

N Liberty St

N Charles St

St Paul Pl

N Calvert St

Guilford Ave

N Gay St

SHOT TOWER PARK

E Baltimore St

Watson St

S High St

E Lombard St

W Fayette St

Carroll Museum

W Baltimore St

W Lombard St

Light St

S Calvert St

South St

Commerce St

S Gay St

HOLOCAUST MEMORIAL PARK

S President St

Star-Spangled Banner Flag House

S Exeter St

Stiles St

Fawn St

Edward A. Garmatz Courthouse

Transamerica Bank of Tower America Center

W Pratt St

E Pratt St

Power Plant Building

Miss Shirley's Café

McKeldin Square

Pratt Street Pavilion

World Trade Center

Columbus Center

Trinity St

Sports Legends Museum

Baltimore Convention Center

S Charles St

USS Constellation

Lightship Chesapeake

U.S. Coast Guard Cutter Taney

COLUMBUS PARK

President Street Station

Harborplace

National Aquarium

Public Works Museum

Fleet St

Camden Station

E Conway St

Baltimore Visitor Center

USS Torsk

finish

start

S Sharp St

Chesapeake Bay

Light St

E Lee St

Maryland Science Center

RASH FIELD

E Lee St

Key Hwy

FEDERAL HILL PARK

0 200 400 600 feet

0 100 200 300 meters

11 CIVIL War Trail: PATH OF THE War's FIRST BLOODSHED

BOUNDARIES: **S. President St., E. Pratt St., S. Howard St.**
DISTANCE: **1.1 miles**
DIFFICULTY: **Easy**
PARKING: **Some street parking on President St. Garage parking off Pratt St. and Howard St.**
PUBLIC TRANSIT: **Light Rail Camden Station/Pratt St. stop. MTA bus #11 runs along President St.; MTA buses #s 7, 10, 11, and 30, and the Charm City Circulator Orange run along Pratt St.; MTA buses #s 120, 160, 320, 410, 411, and 420 all stop at or near Camden Station on Howard St.**

Along this route, you will be following the path of a regiment of Massachusetts volunteers who answered President Abraham Lincoln's call to defend Washington, D.C. Before the Baltimore and Potomac Tunnel was built in 1873, arriving passengers in Baltimore had to come through President Street Station and leave from Camden Station, 10 blocks across town to the west by horsecar. The trip from one to the other on April 19, 1861, saw an escalating skirmish as the Union soldiers fought civilians in the street, shocking the conscience of the nation in a way that the peaceful surrender at Fort Sumter, a week earlier, simply had not. Baltimore was the country's third-largest city at the time; what happened here mattered a great deal to the country at large. This walk requires a bit of imagination, as very little of the landscape those participants saw in 1861 exists today, most of it wiped out by the Great Fire of 1904. But the streets and the city layout are the same, and so you can follow, more or less, the same path as the battle. The route today runs parallel to the Inner Harbor, and so there is much to see, different as it may be from 1861. Nevertheless, squint your eyes the right way and read the interpretative signs along the route and you can just as easily imagine the scene 150 years ago and the indelible mark it left on the city and the country.

Note: Portions of this walk intersect with three other walks in this book: Walk 4: Inner Harbor Promenade, Walk 5: Harbor East, and Walk 13: Downtown: The Raven to the Ravens.

● **Start at President Street Station, 601 S. President St. In addition to its Civil War connections, President Street Station holds an important place in American railroading** history: built in 1849, it remains the country's oldest major city railroad terminal. Today, the station is home to the Baltimore Civil War Museum, run by the Maryland Historical Society. Be sure to go inside to get a sense of how this building played such an integral part in the unfolding story of the Pratt Street Riot.

There were four political factions vying for the presidency in 1860: Abraham Lincoln's Republican Party, plus the northern Democrats, the southern Democrats, and the Constitutional Unionists. The three non-Republican parties all met in Baltimore that year to conduct their nominations. But it was Lincoln's trip to Baltimore a few months later, as President-elect, that helped set the stage for the skirmish on Pratt Street. Rumors of assassination attempts in Baltimore preceded Lincoln's trip through the city on his way to Washington, and so he arrived in the wee hours of the morning and made his way quietly and surreptitiously from one station to the other. One Lincoln contemporary later wrote: "Darkness and silence reigned over all. Perhaps, at this moment, however, the restless conspirators were astir, perfecting their plans for a tragedy as infamous as any which has ever disgraced a free country." Indeed, a Pennsylvania regiment making the same transit on April 18 wasn't so lucky. Southern-sympathizers pelted them with rocks and bricks as they traveled from President Street Station to Camden Station. Fortunately, no one was killed at this time. However, the next day the 6th Massachusetts Volunteer Militia attempted the same trip, and the first blood of the Civil War was shed. When they arrived at President Street Station, on a Friday morning, the regiment's commander, Colonel Edward F. Jones, warned his men to anticipate hostility, saying: "You will undoubtedly be insulted, abused and perhaps assaulted, to which you must pay no attention whatever, but march with your faces square to the front, and pay no attention to the mob, even if they throw stones, bricks, or other missiles; but if you are fired upon, and any of you are hit, your officers will order you to fire. Do not fire into any promiscuous crowds, but select any man whom you may see aiming at you, and be sure you drop him."

● Cross Fleet St., heading north on S. President St. to follow the soldiers' path. Things actually began relatively well; nine trolley cars full of soldiers made it across town to Camden Station, suffering only minor damage from hurled rocks. It was the soldiers following them who ran into trouble.

Look for the extraordinary brick building on your left, just before Eastern Ave. This 1912 still-functioning pumping station was once the home of the fascinating Public Works Museum. When it operated, it was apparently the only public works museum in the world: a massive museum dedicated to sewers, water treatment, and the maze of plumbing operations that exist under the city streets, including a rare 1780s wooden drain pipe. But, like the City Life Museums, Public Works became a victim of shrinking city budgets; hopefully, it will be resurrected when times are more flush. Continue walking north along S. President St. To the left, at E. Falls Ave. and Eastern Ave., is Columbus Park, complete with a series of Italian flags and a beautiful statue of Christopher Columbus, the youngest of the three monuments to Columbus in Baltimore (after Herring Park's 1792 statue and Druid Hill's 1892 memorial).

● Take a left when you reach E. Pratt St. Many locals assume Pratt St. was named for the great city patron Enoch Pratt. But in fact, the street takes its name from Charles Pratt, the 1st Earl of Camden. City maps show Pratt Street appearing as early as 1801. A few blocks north of where you turned stand the Phoenix Shot Tower and St. Vincent de Paul Catholic Church (see Walk 10: Little Italy & Jonestown/Old Town); both would have been visible to the Massachusetts soldiers coming through Baltimore that day; otherwise, the landscape has been completely altered since that time by the Great Fire and subsequent development.

On the corner is Scarlett Place Condominiums, and behind it is the Columbus Center. In between, Pratt St. spans the Jones Falls, here a ribbon of water contained like a canal, heading out to the harbor. In 1861, a wooden bridge spanned the Jones Falls, and it was here that

Pratt St. looking west

Back Story

The role of Baltimore and Maryland is essential to understanding the Civil War. Because of its geographic location south of the Mason-Dixon line, many people assume Maryland was part of the Confederacy. And, indeed, many Marylanders had Southern sympathies. But more residents favored the Union; by sheer numbers, almost three times as many Marylanders fought for the Union than the Confederacy. Additionally, strong federal lobbying efforts persuaded Maryland officials to stay in the Union; otherwise, Washington, D.C., carved out of Maryland land, would be entirely surrounded by the enemy, with neighboring Virginia the capital of the Confederacy. Lincoln recognized Maryland's central place in maintaining the Union, declaring in Baltimore, "Recently, it seems, the people of Maryland have been doing something to define liberty; and thanks to them that, in what they have done, the wolf's dictionary has been repudiated." To this day, Maryland's cultural and political temperaments are far more closely aligned with Northern states than the South. Nevertheless, as another sign of its historical ambivalence, the state song, "Maryland, My Maryland," containing baldly pro-Confederate sentiments, was penned by Baltimorean James Ryder Randall as a reaction to the Pratt Street Riot and includes the reference, "Avenge the patriotic gore / That flecked the streets of Baltimore."

the first shots rang out. Two blocks west, at S. Gay St., the 10th trolley car coming from President Street Station had been stopped. A crowd of men threw sand and heavy anchors across the trolley tracks, disabling the car and causing a bottleneck that delayed the men bringing up the rear. As the growing mob pelted the crippled trolley at Gay St., the Massachusetts men decided to turn around and head back to President Street Station.

These 220 men were quickly surrounded, somewhere near President and Fawn Streets; to escape the barrage of stones, they turned yet again and made it back to Pratt St., where someone—accounts differ—started shooting. The battle was in full rage now, with soldiers firing into the crowd and civilians throwing stones and rushing the soldiers, in some cases seizing their weapons and firing back. The soldiers headed west along Pratt St., where you should continue your walk.

● E. Pratt St. in 1861 was a much narrower street than it is today. What the soldiers saw as they fought their way toward Camden Station would have been wharves along the water's edge to the south, with small businesses—taverns, goods and groceries, and brothels—along the northern side. As you round the corner onto E. Pratt St., you'll find the delectable Miss Shirley's Café on the right and the Institute of Marine and Environmental Technology (IMET), in the old Columbus Center building on the left. IMET is a joint research center involving the University of Maryland, Baltimore County (UMBC); the University of Maryland Center for Environmental Science (UMCES); and the University of Maryland, Baltimore (UMB). The scientists at IMET conduct marine and environmental research. Floating in the water just in front of the marine research center is the U.S. Coast Guard Cutter *Taney*, named for Supreme Court Chief Justice Roger Taney, a Marylander. The ship enjoyed an illustrious military career but derives its fame today primarily from its distinction of being the last ship still afloat that was involved in the Battle of Pearl Harbor. The *Taney* served in both WWII theaters and helped in the search for Amelia Earhart, among other distinctions. She was decommissioned in 1986 and was added to the National Register of Historic Places two years later. Today the *Taney* is part of the collection of the Historic Ships in Baltimore, a maritime museum offering tours of three ships, all National Historic Landmarks, and two lighthouses in and around the harbor. (See "Points of Interest" on page 89 for more information.) Also on the same pier as the *Taney* is the Seven Foot Knoll Lighthouse—for the lowdown, see Walk 4: Inner Harbor Promenade.

● Across the water is the impressive Power Plant building, listed on the National Register of Historic Places in 1987. Its large guitar, heralding the Hard Rock Café inside and attached to a tall smokestack, is a distinctive feature. The country's first ESPN Zone was installed in this building, but it closed in 2010. The building itself was constructed in the first decade of the 20th century and is neoclassical in design. The plant's original function was to supply power to the city's system of electric railways. Later, Baltimore Gas & Electric's predecessor used the power plant as a central steam-supply plant.

● Next up as you travel west is S. Gay St, named for Nicholas Ruxton Gay, who aided in the planning of Baltimore in 1747. Somewhere between here and Light St., four blocks west, is where the Union Army suffered its first casualty of the Civil War. A 17-year-old Massachusetts private named Luther Ladd was shot to death. The exact spot is unknown, so you will find no markers. But if you're still thirsting for history, head toward the water at S. Gay St., to Pier 3, home to the world-famous National Aquarium in Baltimore and the two historic ships docked between the aquarium and the World Trade Center: the Lightship 116 *Chesapeake* and the USS *Torsk.* The aquarium and the ships take you away from the Civil War route, so they are not covered here. However, for specific information on these major attractions, see Walk 4: Inner Harbor Promenade.

● To stay more closely aligned with the skirmish, continue west on Pratt St., where the battle in 1861 was by now at a fever pitch. Though ordered by their commander to be discriminate if pressed to open fire, accounts have it that the Massachusetts soldiers had by this point lost discipline and fought as hard and as wildly as their mobbing adversaries.

A monument to a very different kind of tragedy will be just to your left, in the shadow of the Baltimore World Trade Center. The memorial you see is constructed of three steel beams from the felled twin towers in New York melded with pieces of limestone from the Pentagon's west wall. On September 11, 2001, 68 Marylanders lost their lives, so the memorial here is apt. The building itself holds the distinction of being the world's tallest pentagonal building. You can enjoy sweeping views of Baltimore from the observation deck on the 27th floor.

● Continue west, passing Commerce St. (If you peek northward up Commerce St., you'll catch a glimpse of the lovely, redbrick Chamber of Commerce building, built immediately after the Great Fire of 1904. It's on the National Register of Historic Places.) To your left is the Pratt Street Pavilion, one of two major waterside collections of shops and restaurants, essential in Baltimore's late-20th-century renaissance. A century or two earlier, what you would have seen instead were oyster fleets, docks, and wharves, jam-packed with men making a trade in the Chesapeake's bounty. Behind the Pratt Street Pavilion is docked the USS *Constellation,* truly a magnificent ship with an extraordinary history; see Walk 4: Inner Harbor Promenade.

● The next block is South St. Where the Renaissance Harborplace Hotel stands today, at the corner of South and Pratt, is where the Confederacy lost its first recruit. Baltimore native William R. Clark had enlisted in the Confederate army just days before and was awaiting movement south when he was killed at this spot.

● Just ahead is the intersection of Pratt St. and Light St., where the fighting intensified even further. William Reed, a boy aboard an oyster boat near where the *Constellation* is docked today, was killed by a stray bullet. Another boy, Patrick Griffin, was "shot through the bowels while looking through [a] door," and killed, according to the *Baltimore Sun.*

● Continue on Pratt St., crossing Light St., and passing McKeldin Square, with its decorative fountains, on your left. This is the location taken over by Occupy Baltimore, part of the Occupy Wall Street movement, for almost three months at the end of 2011. This strip is part of Baltimore's commercial heart, evidenced by one commercial building after another. Just to your right is 100 E. Pratt, a building distinctive for its 100,000-plus-square-foot glass and metal tower.

● When you approach the corner of Light St. and Pratt St., at the edge of McKeldin Square, you can take a few steps to your left, where you'll see a "Civil War Trails" sign and an informational panel detailing the events of the Pratt Street Riot.

● Return to Pratt St. and cross Light St. (don't be confused by having already crossed Light once before, as the road splits at Pratt and takes up at slightly different places without contiguity). Pass on the right the Transamerica Tower, which was built as the USF&G building and was known locally for years as the Legg Mason building for the Legg Mason lettering just below the roof. At 40 stories, it's downtown's tallest building, the tallest in Maryland, and the tallest in the Mid-Atlantic south of Philadelphia and north of Raleigh. Light St. heading north, as well as the surrounding blocks, has a host of some of Baltimore's most distinctive downtown buildings and monuments, some of which you can see from this vantage point. But these are covered in Walk 12: Downtown: Contrasts.

During the riot, Police Marshal George P. Kane erected a line of officers in this area, separating the Massachusetts soldiers and Baltimore civilians, hoping to stave off further casualties. Kane, as well as Mayor George W. Brown, were both Southern-sympathizers. But each was desperate to keep the streets of Baltimore free of blood. Eventually, both the mayor and the police commissioner were detained at Fort McHenry for their Confederate sympathies.

- Cross Charles St., where you'll see the 18-story Bank of America Center ahead to the right. Limestone fountains bisecting the sidewalk mark the spot. This and other near-by buildings will be recognizable to anyone who has ever caught an Orioles game at Camden Yards, as each of these peeps over the outfield bleachers. To your left is the north side of the Baltimore Convention Center, opened in 1979 and renovated in 1996–97, and boasting more than 1.25 million square feet of convention space. The gatherings it hosts in any given year are as eclectic as the city itself, but one annual draw that thoroughly transforms downtown is Otakon, a celebration of anime, manga, and all facets of Asian pop culture. Its participants don wildly excessive costumes and parade around downtown to amused gawks. The convention center sprawls over two blocks, bisected by Sharp St.

- Pass S. Hanover St., and the next block is Hopkins Pl., where on the corner is the Edward A. Garmatz Courthouse, named for the US Representative for Maryland from 1947 to 1973; he was Thomas D'Alesandro Jr.'s replacement to Congress when the latter resigned his seat to become mayor of Baltimore. The building houses the US District Court, a US Bankruptcy Court, and a US Court of Appeals. In front of the building is a statue of Thurgood Marshall, the Baltimore native who was the country's first African American Supreme Court Justice (see Walk 17: Pennsylvania Avenue).

- You'll see the distinctive staircase-top office building on your right at the cor-ner of Pratt and S. Howard St. Howard St. is one of three in Baltimore named for Revolutionary War hero John Eager Howard (the other two being Eager St. and John St.). Here is where the Massachusetts regiment turned south, down Howard St., toward Camden Station. You'll notice the Light Rail tracks at Howard St. Follow them south. With the convention center on your left, you'll see Camden Station ahead on your right.

- Cross W. Camden St. to Camden Station, your final destination. Camden Station was built in 1856 and was at the time Baltimore's tallest building. Adjacent to Camden Station is Oriole Park at Camden Yards, a magnificent stadium. (See Walk 13:

Downtown: The Raven to the Ravens for a complete description of the stadium and its history.)

As noted above, President Lincoln came to Camden Station several times, the first being his low-profile escape across town in early 1861. He also passed through on his way to Gettysburg, where he delivered his famous address. His last trip was after his murder; his body lay here for public viewing and dedication. Camden Station also saw a major labor uprising against the B&O in 1877—15,000 workers protested by tearing up tracks, lighting fires, and stoning an engine. Many labor historians consider the strike the beginning of the modern labor movement. Of course, it also contributed to Baltimore's reputation and erstwhile nickname, "Mobtown."

Today, Camden Station no longer functions as a rail depot, but instead houses two museums. The Sports Legends Museum contains an exhaustive display of Maryland sports memorabilia—Ruth, Unitas, Colts, Orioles, Ravens, and much more. The second museum is the unique Geppi's Entertainment Museum, dedicated to telling the story of the history of popular culture. Kids will love it; adults will be socked with some serious nostalgia. There's a particular focus on comic books, but the museum displays all manner of childhood distractions, segregated by room and era, from the 1890s to the present.

By the time the Massachusetts regiment made it to Camden Station, under the protection of police, Colonel Jones made the wrenching decision to leave behind those of his men who had been killed or wounded and lit out for Washington before the mob could block the tracks. The final death occurred a quarter mile south; as the train left Baltimore, a soldier on board fired into a crowd shouting pro-Southern epithets. Local Robert W. Davis died from the shot, further inflaming the mob, who then destroyed the bridges into town to prevent more Northern troops from arriving.

The riot proved a touchstone for both North and South. Many Northerners called for the destruction of Baltimore. President Lincoln helped to defuse tensions by receiving federal troop reinforcements for Washington through Annapolis and promising city leaders that no more troops would come through Baltimore in the immediate future. Despite the riot in the streets and the civilian deaths, the Maryland General Assembly overwhelmingly voted down a resolution to join the secession. Many of the state's most enthusiastic Confederate-sympathizers soon moved to Virginia and things more or less settled down in Baltimore, excepting a few minor disturbances between police and civilians. Nevertheless, General Benjamin Butler stationed 500 Union troops atop Federal Hill on May 13; surviving images show cannons trained on the city below. Some of the troops stationed on Federal Hill were veterans of the Pratt Street Riot.

Somewhat amazingly, President Lincoln was back in Baltimore almost exactly three years later and was well received, basking in a 20-minute ovation. "As soon as he made his appearance he was saluted by cheers," the *Sun* reported. He came once again through Camden Station to give a speech to the Sanitary Fair Commission and visited the Ladies Union Relief Association, an organization created to raise funds for wounded Union soldiers. "Ladies and Gentleman," Lincoln said, "Calling to mind that we are in Baltimore, we cannot fail to note that the world moves. Looking upon these many people, assembled here to serve, as they best may, the soldiers of the Union, it occurs at once that three years ago, the same soldiers could not so much as pass through Baltimore. The change from then till now is both great, and gratifying. Blessings on the brave men who have wrought the change, and the fair women who strive to reward them for it."

The Republican Convention of 1864 was held in Baltimore and Lincoln, in absentia, was renominated for the presidency. He was once again in Baltimore the following year, when his funeral train stopped here on the way home to Illinois.

● From Camden Station, there are a ton of things to do nearby. My recommendation is to cross S. Howard St. to the convention center and follow the sidewalk around the center to the first left onto W. Conway St. At the next block, S. Sharp St., you'll see one of the older buildings in the immediate area: the still-functioning Old Otterbein Church, "the mother church of the United Brethren in Christ and the oldest church edifice in continuous use in the city of Baltimore" (oldotterbeinumc.org). The church was built in 1785 and was named for Philip William Otterbein, a German missionary to Pennsylvania colonists who came to Baltimore in 1774 and stayed until his death in 1813. The parsonage, also on site, was built in 1811.

● To return to your starting point across the harbor, link up with Walk 4: Inner Harbor Promenade by continuing south on W. Conway St. three and a half blocks straight to the harbor and the Baltimore Visitor Center. Go inside for loads of great tourist (and local) information, and then stroll the harbor back around toward President Street Station.

POINTS OF INTEREST (START TO FINISH)

President Street Station/Baltimore Civil War Museum 601 President St., 443-220-0290

Historic Ships in Baltimore historicships.org, 301 E. Pratt St.

Top of the World Observation Level viewbaltimore.org, 401 E. Pratt St., 27th floor, 410-837-VIEW

Geppi's Entertainment Museum geppismuseum.com, 301 W. Camden St., 410-625-7060

Sports Legends Museum baberuthmuseum.com/history/slmacy, 301 W. Camden St., 410-727-1539

Old Otterbein United Methodist Church oldotterbeinumc.org, 112 W. Conway St., 410-685-4703

ROUTE SUMMARY

1. Start at President Street Station, 601 S. President St. and go north.
2. Turn left onto E. Pratt St.
3. Turn left onto S. Howard St. to Camden Station.

CONNECTING THE WALKS

As noted, three walks intersect with this one: Walk 4: Inner Harbor Promenade, Walk 5: Harbor East, and Walk 13: Downtown: The Raven to the Ravens.

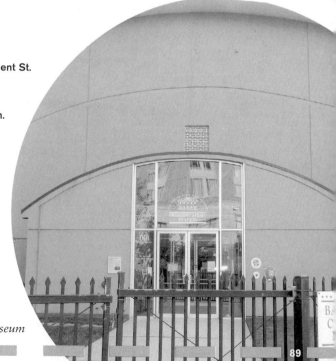

Baltimore Civil War Museum

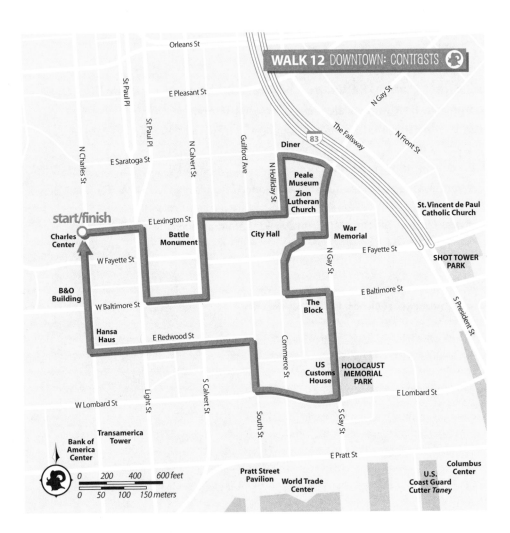

WALK 12 DOWNTOWN: CONTRASTS

Orleans St

E Pleasant St

St Paul Pl

E Saratoga St

St Paul Pl

N Charles St

N Calvert St

Guilford Ave

N Holliday St

Diner

83

The Fallsway

N Gay St

N Front St

Peale Museum

Zion Lutheran Church

St. Vincent de Paul Catholic Church

start/finish

E Lexington St

Battle Monument

City Hall

War Memorial

E Fayette St

SHOT TOWER PARK

Charles Center

W Fayette St

N Gay St

E Baltimore St

S President St

B&O Building

W Baltimore St

The Block

Hansa Haus

E Redwood St

Commerce St

US Customs House

HOLOCAUST MEMORIAL PARK

E Lombard St

W Lombard St

Light St

S Calvert St

South St

S Gay St

Bank of America Center

Transamerica Tower

E Pratt St

Columbus Center

0   200   400   600 feet

0   50   100   150 meters

Pratt Street Pavilion

World Trade Center

U.S. Coast Guard Cutter Taney

12 DOWNTOWN: Contrasts

BOUNDARIES: **N. Charles St., Saratoga St., Gay St., E. Lombard St.**
DISTANCE: **1.5 miles**
DIFFICULTY: **Moderate**
PARKING: **Street parking all along route, but metered and often difficult to obtain in the financial district. Parking garages are also available along route.**
PUBLIC TRANSIT: **Metro stops at Charles Center S/B and Charles Center N/B; MTA buses #s 1, 5, 8, 10, 20, 23, 30, 36, 40, 46, 48, 91, and 120 all stop at Charles Center Metro; most stop at Gay and Lexington as well. MTA bus #15 stops at Lexington and Guilford; MTA buses #s 5, 8, 20, 23, 30, 35, 36, 91, 150, and 160 all stop at Calvert and Fayette. MTA buses #s 1, 61, 64, 120, 310, 410, and 411 all stop at Redwood and Light. The Charm City Circulator Orange and Purple routes intersect with this walk.**

This walk has a stunning array of sites and perfectly encapsulates the great contrasts that contribute to making Charm City truly unique. Starting in what is considered the center of Baltimore (where streets gain their identifier: east, west, north, or south) and in the path of the original 1729 plans for Baltimore-Town, this walk moves away from the financial district, taking in buildings new and old, those that survived the Great Fire of 1904 and those that didn't (plus some that still bear the scars), and an embarrassment of historical riches. These are the sights just north of the Inner Harbor, in an area where few tourists venture. Pity that, as a walk down these streets gives one a sense of what Baltimore used to be and what it is today. The contrasts here are enormous: stately City Hall, the sobering Holocaust Memorial, the adult attractions of the Block, and much, much more. Truly one of the great walks and a great way to appreciate The Monumental City.

● Start on the corner of N. Charles St. and Lexington St. At 100 N. Charles is One Charles Center, a 1962 skyscraper that was the cornerstone of downtown urban renewal. Many locals still lament the modern bent of this building. But the present energy is palpable here in Baltimore's financial district; busy workers scurrying back and forth, all contributing to the local economy. True, there were older and far more beautiful buildings that stood here before Charles Center. But just look in all directions; you'll see plenty of downtown's older buildings still intact. One of them is right across Lexington St. on the northwest corner. This is the lovely Romanesque Revival flatiron-shaped Fidelity & Deposit Company building. This 1890s building was one of the few in the immediate area to survive the Great Fire of 1904. The damage totaled more than $150 million, and that's in 1904 dollars. Give yourself some distance from the front of the building to pick out an amazing sight: if you look closely, you can see the façade of the original 19th-century building's eight floors. Between 1912 and 1915, workers built around it, almost perfectly incorporating all the design elements of the original, expanding it by seven stories.

Head east on E. Lexington St., away from Charles Center, taking in the lovely brick and stone façades of the buildings lining the south side of Lexington. At the end of the block, turn right onto St. Paul St., looking toward the harbor. Across St. Paul is the Greek Revival Clarence Mitchell Courthouse, built between 1896 and 1900 and bearing the name of the local Civil Rights leader since 1985.

In front of the courthouse is the bronze statue of Cecilius Calvert, 2nd Lord Baltimore (1605–1675). Cecilius was the son of George Calvert, the 1st Lord Baltimore. When George died in 1632, Cecilius gained the proprietorship of the colony of Maryland. The statue dates to 1908. The black and gold in Maryland's distinctive state flag is adapted from the Calvert family coat of arms.

Continue heading south on St. Paul St. The first block is Fayette St. Take a quick right here to see two more buildings that date to the rebuilding effort launched in the aftermath of the Great Fire. The Macht building at 15 E. Fayette was destroyed in the fire, but what you see here now was built on the original foundation in 1905. Across the street at 22 E. Fayette is the Hotel Junker building, also built around 1905. Check out the exquisite stonework on these buildings, absolute artistic gems in a sea of far less attractive skyscrapers. It is mind-boggling to consider what superb works of art were lost in the fire; downtown used to be a treasure trove of gorgeous buildings. Fortunately, there are still quite a few worthy of deep admiration, and the Junker and Macht are just two examples. You'll see plenty more on this walk.

Head back to St. Paul and take a right; look for the interesting building at 6 St. Paul. Its distinctive flagpole tower makes it one of the signature points along Baltimore's skyline. This is the William Donald Schaefer Tower; if the flagpole were included, it would be the city's (indeed, the state's) tallest building. Alas, without it, it is only third, at 37 stories. Directly across the street is the 24-story Wachovia Tower, in the top 20 of the city's tallest buildings.

● When you come to the next block, Baltimore St., St. Paul turns to Light St. The next building on the right is an absolute beauty—a skyscraper as it should be. This 37-story Art Deco, brick-and-stone building is the Bank of America building (formerly the Baltimore Trust Company building and the Maryland National Bank building). When it was constructed in 1929–30, it was the state's tallest building and the tallest office building in the country south of New York. If you can situate yourself properly, look up to see beyond the soaring gorgeousness of the lower, middle, and upper floors to the distinctive copper and gold roof. Along the way, spot the Mayan statues and reliefs above and around the entranceway. Pop inside to see the beautiful lobby too, to check out the murals inside depicting the Great Fire (and God protecting the Baltimore Trust Bank), the Battle of Baltimore, and the writing of the national anthem.

● Turn around, return to Baltimore St., and go right (east). As you move down Baltimore St., you'll see more of the same: the skyscrapers of the financial district mingling with some of the fancy façades of the district's older buildings. Baltimore St. was one of the first streets laid out in Baltimore-Town. It initially had other names, including Long St. and Market St. But the name Baltimore St. dates to at least 1745.

● Proceed to the next block: Baltimore St. and N. Calvert St. While this intersection doesn't retain any 18th-century structures, it is actually the oldest developed corner in the city; in fact, Calvert was the name given this street in 1729 and it has remained so all these years—the only such street in the original 18th-century

Old B&O Building

plan. There is one important historic building still on this corner: at 135 E. Baltimore is the former headquarters of Alex Brown Inc., the country's first investment bank, founded in 1800. This two-story brick building, constructed in 1901, is one of the area buildings to survive the Great Fire and was the first building in the country to be heated entirely by electricity. The building's survival was due primarily to the brick and granite construction materials on the façade. Other banks took note, and in following years, a proliferation of similarly styled banks popped up all over the city. Today, Chevy Chase Bank inhabits the space. Take a close look at the large metal doors; they still bear the dents and scars from the fire. If you go inside, look up to see the gorgeous stained glass ceiling, which was restored in 1997. Across Calvert is the 1900–01 Continental Trust building, which also survived the fire. The writer Dashiell Hammett (*The Maltese Falcon*) worked for many years for the Pinkerton Detective Agency in this building.

● Take a left onto N. Calvert, where you'll immediately see two more historic buildings facing each other on opposite sides of the street. On the right is the Equitable building, at 10 N. Calvert, designed in 1889 by local architect Joseph Evans Sperry; it was considered the city's first commercial skyscraper. Its cast-iron and steel girder construction allowed the exterior to survive the fire. (The interior was largely destroyed but soon rebuilt.) Barnum's Hotel stood here before the Equitable, from 1825 to 1889, and was known as an extremely civilized place. Charles Dickens, staying there in 1842, called it "the most comfortable of all hotels in the United States." The hotel's register showed the signatures of many famous guests: John Wilkes Booth, James Buchanan, Stephen Douglas, Cyrus McCormick, Samuel Morse, Charles Lewis Tiffany, Eli Whitney, plus many of the principals of John Brown's raid on Harpers Ferry and hundreds of Civil War soldiers and officers from both sides of the conflict. Seeking to retain the splendorous legacy of the hotel it replaced, the Equitable contained not only offices, but also a billiard parlor, a rooftop garden, a basement barber shop, and Turkish baths.

Across from the Equitable is the Munsey building (1911) at 7 N. Calvert. It was Baltimore's tallest office building when it was completed and carries the name of its original owner, newspaper magnate Frank Munsey.

● Continue north on N. Calvert and you'll immediately come to one of Baltimore's great and unique monuments, the Battle Monument. The monument commemorates those who died defending Baltimore from the British in the War of 1812. Its construction began in 1815 on the site of what had been Baltimore's first courthouse in the 1700s. The courthouse remained until 1800, when it was razed and a new courthouse built on the west side of Calvert. French architect Maximilian Godefroy (see Walk 18: Seton Hill & Lexington Market) designed the monument, giving it two bas-reliefs depicting the battles at North Point and Fort McHenry.

What is striking about this monument's significance (apart from its beauty) is its nod to the "common man." This was the country's first public monument, and it is believed to be the world's first memorial erected in honor of the everyday soldier; to that point, battle monuments had depicted the elite officer and largely ignored the grunt fighter. Reflecting the immense satisfaction the city felt for its citizen soldiers and the singular role they played in defending the young country gives Baltimoreans a sense of real pride to this day. Indeed, this monument sits in the middle of the field of yellow and black in the Baltimore city flag and has been the city's official symbol since 1827. Look closely and you will see the names of the 39 soldiers who died in the conflict on the bands that circle the column, this atop 18 layers of stone—one layer for each of the states in the Union in 1814, when the Baltimore battles took place.

Atop the column stands the regal Lady Baltimore holding a victory wreath. You will no doubt also see that Lady Baltimore has sustained some damage in her almost 200 years atop her column. A straight shot to the harbor, bad weather has been racing off the water and up Calvert right into the monument since its beginning. In 2012, city officials devised a plan to have a replica made and put in her place; the original will find a home in the Walters Art Museum (see Walk 16: Mount Vernon). She deserves a rest, as she has seen her share of history: President John Quincy Adams toasted the monument and thereafter dubbed Baltimore The Monumental City; when President Zachary Taylor put out a call for citizens to fight in the Mexican-American War, volunteers queued up here; and Frederick Douglass gave a speech here after the ratification of the 15th Amendment.

To the right of the Battle Monument is the old United States Post Office and Courthouse building. This 1932 building has seen its share of legal history. Here, Vice President, former Baltimore County executive, and Maryland Governor Spiro Agnew pleaded no contest to tax evasion and resigned his office; alleged Soviet spy and local

Alger Hiss filed a libel lawsuit against his public accuser, Whittaker Chambers, in a case that took the country by storm in 1948; and in the late 1960s, the Berrigan brothers—Philip and Daniel—peace activists and part of the Catonsville Nine (convicted of entering a Catonsville, Maryland, draft board and burning almost 400 draft files using homemade napalm, making national news) were indicted in this building. This is actually the second post office building to occupy the site; the first was a gorgeous Italian Renaissance building constructed in 1889. During the Great Fire, post office employees stood above every window and poured water down each using bucket brigades. To this day, the building is a hub of activity, and it's common to see television news cameras out front. It's now known as Courthouse East and has been listed on the National Register of Historic Places since 1977.

● Go to the end of the block and take a right onto E. Lexington St. at the Court Square building (1929)—ornate designs above the 2nd and 18th floors have much in common with the monument below. Go three blocks to N. Holliday St. (no connection to Billie Holiday, but instead named for John Holliday, Baltimore sheriff in 1770), passing City Hall on your right—you'll return to City Hall soon. Go left onto N. Holliday. On the corner of Lexington and Holliday is the redbrick Zion Lutheran Church. This is the state's oldest Lutheran congregation, founded in 1755. The church you see now was built in pieces over many years. But the oldest sections date to 1807. Unfortunately, the bulk of that structure burned in 1840, but the church was rebuilt soon after. The tower and parish hall date to 1912. This is a bilingual church, and services are conducted in German, as they have been for more than 200 years.

● Continue north on N. Holliday. The next building ahead to the right is the Peale Museum building. Sadly, it no longer functions in its original capacity. But its very presence is a testament to an amazing story. In 1814, the famed portrait painter Rembrandt Peale (among his subjects were George Washington and Thomas Jefferson) built this structure and opened Peale's Baltimore Museum and Gallery of Fine Arts, making it the first structure built in the Western Hemisphere designed solely as a museum. Among many portraits, including his own creations, Peale exhibited a complete mastodon skeleton, exhumed by his father Charles Wilson Peale, also a renowned portraitist, in 1801. The collections grew, and soon enough animal and ethnographic pieces far outnumbered portraits. The museum hung on until 1830, when it was sold and its contents moved. Subsequently, the building served as the first City Hall of Baltimore (1830–1875) and later operated as the Number 1 Colored Primary School. By the late 20th century, local civic leaders and preservationists restored it to its original function, and it eventually became part of the wonderful and long-mourned City Life Museums in 1985. Now, sadly, it has lost its life as a museum; closed in 1997, it awaits resurrection. Much of the museum's contents are safely stored with the Maryland Historical Society (see Walk 16: Mount Vernon). The name is still there, however: look above the lintel to see the carved words, "Municipal Museum of the City of Baltimore."

● Facing the building, go down the alley that separates the Peale from the Zion Lutheran Church grounds. Take a peek over the wall to your left into the Peale Museum courtyard for a fascinating treat. There, you will find massive slabs of early 19th-century artwork salvaged from area buildings that were razed. The biggest one depicts Ceres and Neptune flanking the Maryland coat of arms; it once decorated the façade of the Union Bank building. It is more than 200 years old, making it one of the oldest pieces of building sculpture in the country.

● After returning to N. Holliday, continue north. At the next intersection, Saratoga St., take a right, but not before checking out the lonely-looking diner across Saratoga. Fans of the 1982 Barry Levinson movie *Diner* will instantly recognize the place. (It also had a prominent role in Levinson's *Tin Men*.) Yes, this is the same diner as the one in the movie, then taken from a salvage yard in New Jersey and planted waterside in Fells Point. Newcomers to Baltimore would do well to watch *Diner* to get a sense of the city (more than 30 years later, locals still love to tell about the famous Colts quiz, administered to Steve Guttenberg's character's fiancée; he will marry her only if she passes the

Battle Monument

grueling test). The movie itself is a delight and launched the careers of many actors who went on to stardom: Ellen Barkin, Kevin Bacon, Steve Guttenberg, Daniel Stern, Mickey Rourke, Tim Daly. The diner has served as an actual restaurant over the years. Check it out to see if it's still operating.

- After taking a right onto Saratoga St., take another right at the next block, N. Gay St. You'll pass the other side of the Zion Lutheran Church on your right before emerging onto a wonderful plaza. Don't miss the Firefighters' Memorial on the corner of N. Gay and E. Lexington, just beyond the church and just before War Memorial Plaza. The monument is relatively new, dating from 1990.

To your left is the stunning War Memorial, instantly recognizable by its three sets of golden double doors and six Doric columns flanked by two sculpted stone horses fording water (signifying American aid to allies overseas). It was built in 1925 to honor Maryland veterans of World War I. A rededication of the building took place in 1977 to honor Marylanders who died in all wars, including and after World War I.

Predating the War Memorial building on this spot was the Holliday Street Theatre, dating to 1794, a famous place that was in its day the country's second-oldest theater. The great Shakespearean actor (and father of John Wilkes Booth) Junius Brutus Booth made his first American appearance in the Holliday Street Theatre. (Booth is one of many luminaries now buried in Greenmount Cemetery; see Walk 21: Station North.) A performance of Francis Scott Key's "Star-Spangled Banner" premiered here too.

- On the west side of War Memorial Plaza is Baltimore City Hall. The construction of this grand old French Revival building dates to the years just after the end of the Civil War. Its mansards, rotunda, grand staircase, and arched windows supported by perfect columns make this building one of the more prominent and stately around—as it should be, housing the mayor and serving as the city's primary seat of government. It hasn't been cheap: when it was built in the 1860s and 1870s, it cost more than $2 million (in 19th-century dollars). Its renovation in the 1970s cost another $10.5 million. But it's a beautiful building, and the choice to renovate the grande dame at great cost instead of razing and building anew was a wise one. Head inside to see the interior, making sure to see the stained glass dome, dominated by an image of the Battle Monument.

In front of City Hall and facing the War Memorial building is the 1972 monument to African American soldiers who died in the service of their country. Nearby, President-elect Obama gave a speech that packed the plaza less than two weeks before he was sworn in as president.

● Head south on N. Holliday St. When you reach the next block, Baltimore St., look for the gas lamp at the northwest corner of the intersection. This replica lamp celebrates the first gas lamp lit in the United States. Peale used one to attract visitors to his museum in 1816, and in a country where all nighttime light came from candles, it proved a sensation. Soon after, Baltimore became the first American city with gas streetlights.

● Take a left onto E. Baltimore. What faces you now is not for the faint of heart: Baltimore's famous Block. This collection of strip clubs and other adult entertainment outlets has been around for almost 100 years, gaining notoriety in the first half of the 20th century as perhaps the East Coast's preeminent center for burlesque houses. Pulitzer Prize–winning Baltimore writer Russell Baker wrote of the Block: "When strip-tease still seemed vital, it was one of the earth's cultural centers." Many of burlesque's most famous entertainers, including Blaze Starr, got their start here. But as the burlesque houses turned to sex clubs, and prostitution and drug dealing increased, many civic leaders wanted to shut down the area. After all, its location is a curious one, so close to City Hall, the Holocaust Memorial, and more recently a central police station. But all attempts have failed, in large part because Baltimoreans are by and large a live-and-let-live populace. Besides, the thinking goes, if these businesses are contained here in one block, they are easier to manage and oversee. In the end, this is just one more example of local flavor.

● Proceed to the next block, S. Gay St., and take a right. Cross the next block, Water St., and you will find yourself between two more points of interest. On your right is the United States Custom House building. On the National Register of Historic Places since 1974, this Beaux Arts building dates to 1903. This is actually Baltimore's third customhouse (the first two dating to the late 18th and early 19th centuries). The Great Fire swept through as the building was still under construction, and it sustained heavy damage. But parts of the building were salvaged and rebuilt, and it was completed in 1907. Go inside and check out the exquisite Call Room, full of paintings and architecture with nautical themes, a nod to Baltimore's waterside location.

On the other side of Gay St. is the Holocaust Memorial. It's an arresting memorial, taking up an entire block. At the far end, away from Lombard St., are large stones resembling a train. Along the train are the words of a Holocaust survivor, "On both sides of the track rows of red and white lights appeared as far as the eye could see . . . with the rhythm of the wheels, with every human sound now silenced, we awaited what was to happen . . . in an instant, our women, our parents, our children disappeared. We saw them for a short while as an obscure mass at the end of the other end of the platform; then we saw nothing more." In the middle of the plaza is a bronze memorial in the shape of a flame engulfing human bodies wrapped with the words, "Those who cannot remember the past are condemned to repeat it."

- After this sobering place, continue south to E. Lombard St. and take a right. Go one block to South St. and take a right. On the right, at 19–21 South St., is the Furness House, a beautiful building designed in 1917 and named for Sir Christopher Furness, who established a successful shipping company in 1891. Just ahead is the 31-story Commerce Place building, the city's fourth tallest.

- Across from the Furness House, take a left onto E. Redwood St. The building at the corner of Redwood and South is the Garrett building, built in 1913 for the venerable Garrett railroading family. (You can see "Robert Garrett And Sons" etched above the entrance on E. Redwood.) A little farther up the block on the right, at 200 E. Redwood, is the beautiful redbrick Mercantile Deposit & Trust Co. building. The former bank building was built in 1885. The Chesapeake Shakespeare Company acquired the building in 2012 and plans to re-create the Globe Theatre inside, adding an essential element to Baltimore's already thriving and varied theater scene. Stay tuned.

- Go another three blocks west to Charles St. At the corner of Charles and Redwood is the Tudor Hansa Haus. This unique building—so very different from all of its neighbors—was built in 1912 to house the headquarters of the North German Lloyd and Hamburg American steamship lines. The model for the building was the 17th-century courthouse in Halberstadt, Germany. German influence in the area was strong; in fact, before World War I, Redwood Street was actually named German Street. The Hansa Haus served then as a German consulate. Wartime realities led Baltimoreans to scrap the reference to Germany, but fortunately the building survived. (Hanover Street, in South Baltimore, still survives, however.)

● When you emerge onto S. Charles St., you'll be facing the back of the venerable Morris Mechanic Theater. The Mechanic, as it is known to locals, fills Baltimoreans with ambivalence. Many of us have seen some great shows here, and some great actors—Katharine Hepburn and George C. Scott among them—but you'd be hard-pressed to find anyone who actually likes the building itself (though, of course, this being Baltimore, you will certainly find folks all too eager to defend its hideousness). It was built in 1967 in the brutalist style of modernist architecture. With other venues for Broadway shows in town and with the reopening of the beautiful Hippodrome (see Walk 13: Downtown: The Raven to the Ravens), the Mechanic quickly became obsolete, shutting down for good in 2004. Since that time, a fight has raged between preservationists seeking to save the Mechanic with a historic designation and developers ready to tear it down and replace it with residential and commercial properties. This is a terrific location, after all. Whatever happens, one hopes it's a good result, something more positive than the indignity the building suffered in 2009 when Britain's Daily Mail online named it to the top spot on its countdown of the world's Top Ten Ugliest Buildings.

A far more attractive building is just to your right, at the corner of Charles and Baltimore Streets. The Savings Bank of Baltimore building is a Beaux Arts stunner with Greek influences built in 1907. This is in some respects the center of Baltimore. Here, streets are designated east, west, north, or south starting on this block.

● As you continue north on Charles St. (now *North* Charles St.), you'll see catty-corner from the Savings Bank building the even more beautiful B&O Building (now a Hotel Monaco). Headquarters to the great railroading

Firefighters' Memorial, with City Hall in background

company, the Beaux Arts building was constructed in 1906. Check out the entrance to this place; it needs no superlatives.

● Continue heading north on N. Charles St. You'll pass on the left the location of what was once the offices of the *Baltimore Sun* before it moved to its current location on Calvert St. Since starting on Light St. in 1837, the newspaper has moved to five different locations in the city during its 175-plus years of existence. A paper with a great history, the *Sun* provided the primary coverage in the 1925 Scopes Monkey Trial, for one. *Sun* publisher Paul Patterson put up the money for Scopes's bail, and the paper paid the fees for his conviction and much of his attorney's fees. H. L. Mencken's scathing coverage of the "imbeciles" in Tennessee gained him some notoriety. It's also worth noting that his coverage introduced two new phrases into the American lexicon, "Monkey Trial" and "Bible Belt."

● One and a half blocks to the north is the starting point to this walk.

POINTS OF INTEREST (START TO FINISH)

Bank of America Building 10 Light St.

Alex Brown Building 135 E. Baltimore St.

Munsey Building 7 N. Calvert St.

Equitable Building 10 N. Calvert St.

Battle Monument Calvert St., between Fayette St. and Lexington St.

Zion Lutheran Church zionbaltimore.org, 400 E. Lexington St., 410-727-3939

Peale Museum 225 N. Holliday St.

Hollywood Diner 400 E. Saratoga St.

War Memorial 101 N. Gay St., 410-396-8013

Baltimore City Hall baltimorecity.gov, 100 N. Holliday St.

Custom House 40 S. Gay St.

Holocaust Memorial E. Lombard St. and S. Gay St.

Mercantile Deposit & Trust Co. Building 200 E. Redwood St.

Hansa Haus E. Redwood and S. Charles Sts.

route summary

1. Start at N. Charles St. and E. Lexington St.
2. Go east on E. Lexington St.
3. Turn right onto St. Paul St.
4. Turn left onto W. Baltimore St.
5. Turn left onto N. Calvert St.
6. Turn right onto E. Lexington St.
7. Turn left onto N. Holliday St.
8. Turn right onto E. Saratoga St.
9. Turn right onto N. Gay St.
10. Cross War Memorial Plaza.
11. Turn south onto N. Holliday St.
12. Turn left onto E. Baltimore St.
13. Turn right onto S. Gay St.
14. Turn right onto E. Lombard St.
15. Turn right onto South St.
16. Turn left onto E. Redwood St.
17. Turn right onto S. Charles St.

Connecting the walks

When this walk reaches E. Lombard St., you can access Walk 11: Civil War Trail by going one block south to Pratt St.

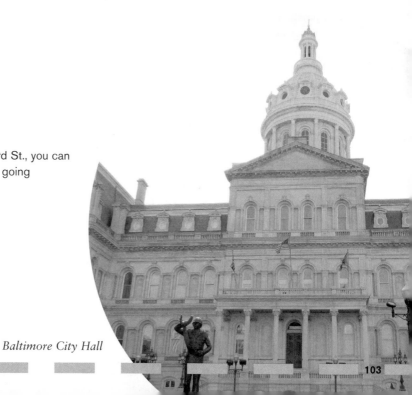

Baltimore City Hall

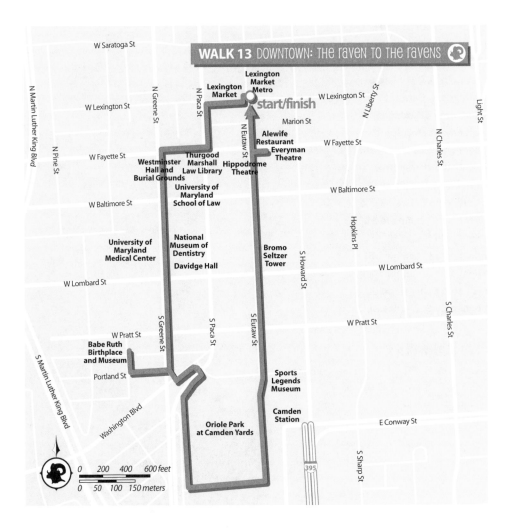

W Saratoga St

N Martin Luther King Blvd

W Lexington St

N Greene St

N Pine St

N Paca St

Lexington Market

Lexington Market Metro

start/finish

W Lexington St

N Liberty St

Marion St

Light St

W Fayette St

Alewife Restaurant

Everyman Theatre

N Charles St

W Fayette St

N Eutaw St

Westminster Hall and Burial Grounds

Thurgood Marshall Law Library

Hippodrome Theatre

University of Maryland School of Law

W Baltimore St

W Baltimore St

University of Maryland Medical Center

National Museum of Dentistry

Davidge Hall

Bromo Seltzer Tower

S Howard St

Hopkins Pl

W Lombard St

W Lombard St

W Pratt St

S Greene St

S Paca St

S Eutaw St

W Pratt St

S Charles St

Babe Ruth Birthplace and Museum

Portland St

Sports Legends Museum

Camden Station

S Martin Luther King Blvd

Washington Blvd

Oriole Park at Camden Yards

395

S Sharp St

E Conway St

0   200   400   600 feet
0   50   100   150 meters

13 DOWNTOWN: The raven to the ravens (and other birds too)

BOUNDARIES: **N. Paca St., W. Lombard St., N. Greene St., S. Greene St., Portland St., Emory St., W. Camden St., S. Eutaw St., N. Eutaw St.**

DISTANCE: **1.6 miles**

DIFFICULTY: **Easy**

PARKING: **Metered street parking along route**

PUBLIC TRANSIT: **Lexington Market Metro, Camden Yards Light Rail, MTA buses #s 1, 7, 8, 17, 19, 20, 27, 30, 35, 36, 40, 46, 48, 91, and 150, and the Charm City Circulator all make stops along the route.**

Downtown is hip. Full of cool sights. But sometimes, even in neighborhoods where those cool sites are concentrated, it's often the case that folks don't string them together. This walk concentrates on quite a few city highlights, but ones that visitors and locals alike rarely see except in isolation. That's because while this section of downtown is a strange and wonderful amalgam of things to see, many of the sites are unrelated to one another. But they're definitely interesting nonetheless. This walk covers many of Baltimore's icons, past and present. It heads through the heart of upper downtown, taking in America's oldest market and first dental school, several museums, the boyhood home of one celebrated native (Babe Ruth) and the final resting place of an adopted son (Edgar Allan Poe), plus restored and rehabbed beauties (the Hippodrome Theatre and the Bromo Seltzer Tower) and stops at what is still the best ballfield in America, Oriole Park at Camden Yards. And then, across the way, you can take in the edifice of Baltimore's newest favorite birds, the Ravens. It's a reminder: downtown is where it's happening.

- Begin at Lexington Market, the oldest continuous market in the United States. For the historical lowdown and what's up at Lexington Market, see Walk 18: Seton Hill & Lexington Market. From Lexington Market, take N. Paca St. south toward W. Fayette St. Paca St. was named for William Paca, a signer of the Declaration of Independence.

- When you reach W. Fayette St., take a right, passing the University of Maryland School of Law and the Thurgood Marshall Law Library. Much of the University of Maryland at

Baltimore campus is dedicated to law and medicine and has been located on this and the surrounding blocks for more than 200 years.

Just up on the left, beyond the Law Library, is Westminster Hall and Burial Grounds, the final resting place of Edgar Allan Poe. The gate on the far edge, just near the intersection with N. Greene St., is where you'll find a monument to the cemetery's most famous denizen. But he's not the only Poe here. His wife (and cousin), Virginia Clemm; mother-in-law (and aunt), Maria Clemm; and a brother and grandfather all rest nearby in a family plot where Edgar was originally buried (see "Back Story" on page 108). Obviously, most visitors come to commune with the great writer, but there are other notables buried at Westminster as well. Many of Maryland's 18th- and 19th-century political luminaries are here, including three early mayors of Baltimore, including the city's first, James Calhoun, as well as Constitution signer James McHenry. The cemetery was established in the 1780s. The grounds are fun to wander around, but try to arrange a tour of the beautiful Gothic church itself. Built in 1852 and no longer in use as a place of worship, the church has been restored to pristine condition and boasts a magnificent 1880s pipe organ. In an effort to leave the existing graves intact, the church was originally built on brick piers, creating catacombs that you can tour (see "Points of Interest" on page 110).

● When you are finished at Westminster Hall, take a left onto N. Greene St. heading south. Up the block to the right is the sprawling University of Maryland Medical Center, so you'll probably see a gaggle of resting docs and nurses as you pass University Park on your left. When you reach 31 S. Greene St., pop into the quirky National Museum of Dentistry—there's more there than you ever cared to know about oral health. Its most famous attraction: George Washington's lower denture. Nope, they weren't made of wood, but of ivory instead. The Washington Gallery also tells the woeful tale of our first president's terrible time with teeth.

Behind the National Museum of Dentistry sits Davidge Hall, constructed in 1812 and named for the first dean of the University of Maryland School of Medicine, Dr. John B. Davidge. It has been used for 200 years as a medical learning facility, making it the oldest such building in the country continuously used for medical education.

● The next block, heading south on S. Greene St., is Lombard St. If you look to the left, you will see the Bromo Seltzer Tower, another Baltimore landmark. For now, continue straight. Your return route will take you past the tower. You'll also notice an abundance of eating options if you're hungry.

- Continue on S. Greene St., passing W. Pratt St., and take a right when you reach Portland St.

- Take the first right onto Emory St. You'll notice baseballs painted on the sidewalk; the reason for this soon becomes obvious. Just up to the right, at 216 Emory St., is the Babe Ruth Birthplace and Museum. This handsome row house is where The Babe was a babe, born here in 1895. It barely escaped demolition in the 1960s, but local efforts emanating from the offices of Mayor Theodore McKeldin saved the structure and it became a shrine in 1974. The museum today is only blocks from Oriole Park at Camden Yards and offers displays on one of America's first truly international sports celebrities. Its location is apropos; it was the Orioles who offered Ruth his first major-league contract when he was only 19. His youth led some of his teammates to refer to him as the owner's "newest babe," and the nickname stuck all the way throughout a Hall of Fame career that left him arguably the greatest player in the history of the game.

- Allow Babe Ruth's life to whet your appetite for more baseball. You no doubt noticed Oriole Park at Camden Yards looming ahead when you turned onto Portland St. Retrace your steps back to S. Greene St. and turn right. Cross Washington Blvd. and circle the magnificent stadium. Built in 1992 to replace the beloved but decrepit Memorial Stadium in Waverly, Camden Yards immediately became a local and national hit. It was the first of the retro stadiums, hearkening back to baseball's good old days. It's also significant that the stadium was built downtown in an era when most professional sports stadiums were being built in suburbs, contributing to pollution, sprawl, and urban decay. You need not be a sports fan to appreciate this beautiful structure or the history surrounding the area: during excavation for the new ballpark, workers discovered a tavern privy and a French flintlock pistol—not terribly surprising considering that French army men camped here before heading to the Battle of Yorktown. Perhaps most striking is the giant B&O Warehouse, built 1899–1905, which looms over the stadium. It's a massive presence: eight stories and almost half a million square feet, which allowed the Baltimore & Ohio Railroad to store some 1,000 carloads of freight. Today it serves as the Orioles' administrative offices.

Back Story

In 1875, a Baltimore schoolteacher decided that the incomparable Edgar Allan Poe was not getting his due. Despite being a beloved figure in France, Poe's own country largely ignored him. And here he was in Baltimore, in a family plot with no headstone and no proper acknowledgment for his accomplishments—inventor of the detective story, a great practitioner of the short story, a wonderful poet. This teacher began a "Pennies for Poe" campaign designed to raise money for a monument. If you visit the memorial today, it's quite likely you'll see some coins on the monument, a nod to that original campaign.

On Poe's birthday, January 19, late at night, for some 60 years an unidentified "Poe Toaster" arrived clad in obscuring clothing and solemnly placed roses and cognac on Poe's grave. This tribute began as early as 1949 and carried on all the way until 2009, when it ended. Speculation as to who the shadowy figure was (or, more accurately, who the figures were, as folks did notice that one year the Poe Toaster inexplicably carried a discernibly different body shape from the previous year) became a great Baltimore pastime. Its abrupt end suggests that the Poe Toaster has joined the legendary author in the murky hereafter.

● Walk around the grounds, sneaking a peek at the legends courtyard, where you will see bronzed statues of Orioles' favorites and Hall of Famers: Eddie Murray, Jim Palmer, Cal Ripken Jr., Brooks Robinson, Frank Robinson, and Earl Weaver. Head toward the Warehouse along Camden St. until you reach Camden Station, home of the Sports Legends Museum. Even if you've had enough of sports already, this building is worth a look anyway. Camden Station is 150 years old and was built as a major terminus for the B&O. President Abraham Lincoln passed through this station several times, his first and last appearances offering a grim closure. He first came through en route to his inauguration in Washington, D.C., but did so in the middle of the night, fearing an assassination attempt. His last time here was after being murdered; his body was laid here for public view and dedication. If you asked most Americans where the first blood of the Civil War was shed, many would answer Fort Sumter. But in fact it was right here, just outside this station. (For the whole story, see Walk 11: Civil War Trail.) Camden Station also saw a major labor uprising against the railroad in 1877—15,000 workers protested by tearing up tracks, lighting fires, and stoning an engine. Many labor historians consider the strike the beginning of the modern labor movement.

There is yet one more museum in this historic Camden complex: the unique Geppi's Entertainment Museum, dedicated to telling the story of the history of popular culture. Kids will love it; adults will be socked with some serious nostalgia. There's a particular focus on comic books, but the museum displays all manner of childhood distractions, segregated by room and era, from the 1890s to the present.

- Looking south from Camden Station down Eutaw St., across the ramps for I-395 and I-95, you'll no doubt notice the looming presence of M&T Bank Stadium. This purple edifice is home to the Ravens, who have managed to erase much of the distaste of the Colts' defection in 1984—well, almost. Named for Poe's most famous poem (and sporting three raven mascots: Edgar, Allan, and Poe), the team supplanted the Orioles in most people's hearts as Baltimore's favorite birds, especially after winning the Super Bowl in 2001. But after the Orioles' successful campaign in 2012 rekindled local memories of Oriole dominance from the 1960s through the 1980s, the O's are once again beloved, making Baltimore a two-bird town.

- Take S. Eutaw St. north away from the stadiums. Cross W. Pratt St. and W. Lombard St., where you'll see the Bromo Seltzer Tower. This tower celebrated its centennial in 2011 and has been a Baltimore landmark since its construction. Its distinctiveness is owed primarily to its architectural uniqueness—well, unique to American cities, in any case. The tower was modeled after the Palazzo Vecchio in Florence, Italy. It was the brainchild of Captain Isaac Emerson, the inventor of Bromo Seltzer, the headache remedy. The tower's most distinctive feature is the massive clock, emblazoned with the letters B-R-O-M-O S-E-L-T-Z-E-R where the numbers would normally be. The clock still functions today. The City of Baltimore has converted the tower into space for studio and visual artists, available by application. While civic boosters are thrilled by this re-use, many locals are still pining for the comeback of the original 50-foot Bromo Seltzer bottle (or at least a replica) that used to revolve on top of the tower. Almost 600 lights illuminated the bottle, and legend has it that one could see it a full 20 miles away.

- Heading north on S. Eutaw St., pass Cider Alley, W. Redwood St., and W. Baltimore St., before arriving at the Hippodrome Theatre. The Hippodrome is one of Baltimore's grand old theaters, an impressive neoclassical edifice designed by the noted theater architect Thomas White Lamb in 1914. Inside, the theater is a swirl of curves and semicircles, a baroque space somewhat at odds with the symmetrical, sharp angles of the massive façade. The Hippodrome gained a national reputation from the 1930s through the 1950s and hosted performances from the likes of Morey Amsterdam, the Andrews Sisters, Jack Benny, Milton Berle, Benny Goodman, Bob Hope, Martha Raye, Dinah Shore, and Red Skelton. Frank Sinatra's first appearance with the Tommy Dorsey Orchestra took place in the Hippodrome. The theater eventually lost some of its luster but managed to function until 1990, when it closed. But now that the Hippodrome has been reborn as part of the France-Merrick Performing Arts Center (the theater has been combined with the Western National Bank building [1887], the Eutaw Savings Bank building [1888], and a newly constructed building), it is once again attracting Broadway shows and nationally touring performances.

Across the street from the Hippodrome is the Alewife Restaurant, a cozy bar and restaurant with homey dark colors and a distinctive drinks menu.

● At the next block, W. Fayette St., take a quick detour to the right to check out the progress at 315 W. Fayette. This is the new home for the Everyman Theatre (see Walk 21: Station North). This building has an interesting performance pedigree. It was built in 1910 and opened as The Empire, originally a vaudeville theater. Later incarnations included a Yiddish theater, a venue for boxing matches, and a burlesque, then known as The Palace. In 1947, when it became a movie house, the Town Theatre, it opened with *It's a Wonderful Life,* and star and director Jimmy Stewart and Frank Capra attended. It closed in 1990 and has now received the restoration and new life it deserves, further contributing to the phoenix-like Westside development.

● Return to N. Eutaw St. and go right; two blocks north is Lexington Market, which spans the block from N. Eutaw St., to where you began, at N. Paca St.

POINTS OF INTEREST (STarT TO FINISH)

Lexington Market lexingtonmarket.com, 400 W. Lexington St., 410-685-6169

Westminster Hall westminsterhall.org, 519 W. Fayette St., 410-706-2072

The Dr. Samuel D. Harris National Museum of Dentistry dentalmuseum.org, 31 S. Greene St., 410-706-0600

Davidge Hall, University of Maryland School of Medicine medschool.umaryland.edu/davidge, 522 W. Lombard St.

The Babe Ruth Birthplace and Museum baberuthmuseum.com, 216 Emory St., 410-727-1539

Geppi's Entertainment Museum geppismuseum.com, 301 W. Camden St., 410-625-7060

Sports Legends Museum baberuthmuseum.com/history/slmacy, 301 W. Camden St., 410-727-1539

Bromo Seltzer Arts Tower bromoseltzertower.com, 21 S. Eutaw St., 443-874-3596

France-Merrick Performing Arts Center/Hippodrome Theatre france-merrickpac.com, 12 N. Eutaw St., 410-837-7400

Alewife Restaurant alewifebaltimore.com, 21 N. Eutaw St., 410-545-5112

route summary

1. Start at Lexington Market.
2. Turn south on N. Paca St.
3. Turn right on W. Fayette St.
4. Turn left on N. Greene St. and continue as it turns into S. Greene St.
5. Turn right on Portland St.
6. Turn right on Emory St.
7. Return to S. Greene St.
8. Cross S. Paca St. to Camden Yards.
9. Go east on W. Camden St.
10. Turn left on S. Eutaw St.
11. Follow S. Eutaw St. as it turns into N. Eutaw St. to Lexington Market.

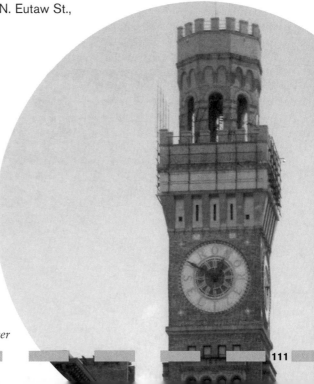

Bromo Seltzer Tower

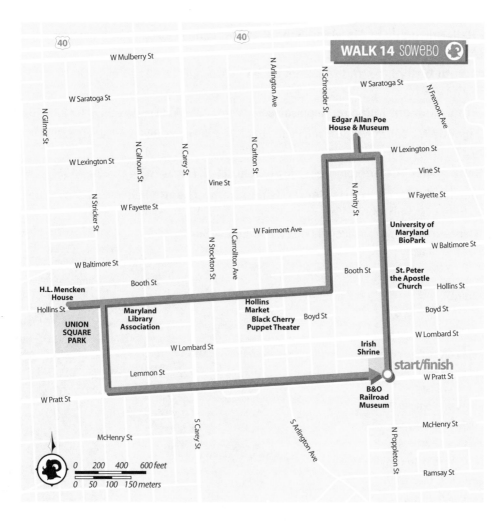

W Mulberry St

W Saratoga St

N Gilmor St

W Lexington St

N Stricker St

W Fayette St

W Baltimore St

H.L. Mencken House

Hollins St

Booth St

UNION SQUARE PARK

Maryland Library Association

Lemmon St

W Pratt St

McHenry St

N Calhoun St

N Carey St

Vine St

N Carrollton Ave

N Stockton St

W Fairmont Ave

Booth St

Hollins Market Black Cherry Puppet Theater

Boyd St

W Lombard St

N Carlton St

N Arlington Ave

N Schroeder St

Edgar Allan Poe House & Museum

W Saratoga St

N Fremont Ave

W Lexington St

Vine St

W Fayette St

N Amity St

University of Maryland BioPark

W Baltimore St

Booth St

St. Peter the Apostle Church

Hollins St

Boyd St

W Lombard St

Irish Shrine

start/finish

W Pratt St

B&O Railroad Museum

S Carey St

S Arlington Ave

N Poppleton St

McHenry St

Ramsay St

0   200   400   600 feet

0   50   100   150 meters

14 SOWEBO: BE IN ON IT

BOUNDARIES: **W. Pratt St., N. Poppleton St., N. Amity St., N. Schroeder St., Hollins St., S. Stricker St.**
DISTANCE: **1.9 miles**
DIFFICULTY: **Moderate**
PARKING: **Street parking along route**
PUBLIC TRANSIT: **MTA buses #10 and #35, and Charm City Circulator Orange**

SOWEBO (Southwest Baltimore) has been struggling to reinvent itself for years. A high crime rate, tenacious poverty, and general hopelessness have long defined some pockets of this area of the city. But things have begun to improve. A vigorous civic association, the arrival on the scene of the new University of Maryland BioPark, and an absolute treasure trove of historical sites make SOWEBO a good place to check out. Visit the sites, walk the streets, patronize local vendors at the annual SOWEBohemian Music & Arts Festival, and be in on the continued revitalization. Your rewards: the homes of two of the most influential writers and thinkers in American literature and letters—Edgar Allan Poe and H. L. Mencken—and the birthplace of American railroading. Not bad for a place many Baltimoreans and outsiders rarely visit.

Note: Some of the areas on this walk have a reputation for crime. If you do this walk on foot, you will pass a lot of urban blight. However, I wish to stress that I've never been bothered or felt unsafe in these neighborhoods, and I believe that the claims of danger are most probably overstated. Nevertheless, exercise common sense and travel during daylight hours. It is possible to do this route by car.

● **Begin at the B&O Railroad Museum. This is one of Baltimore's truly great museums, a real national treasure, containing the oldest and most complete collection of railroading memorabilia in the world. The museum's 40-acre campus is the very site where, in 1829, American railroading was born. The museum boasts in its extensive collection locomotives and other memorabilia from 1830 all the way to the present day. The star attractions are housed in the Mount Clare Station Roundhouse, which was the largest circular industrial building in the world when it was built. Right in the middle of the roundhouse sits the country's first segment of commercial long-distance track. In fact, you can even take a ride on a portion of America's first commercial track just beyond the roundhouse. The U.S. Department of the Interior has** declared the entire museum and its collections a National Historic Landmark, and in 1999 the B&O Museum signed an affiliation agreement with the Smithsonian Institution, the first such museum in the country to be so honored.

Another American (and world) first: it was from here, at Mount Clare Station, that the first telegraph message, announcing the Whig nomination of Henry Clay to the presidency in 1844, was transmitted. Additionally, Henry Morse's famous message, "What hath God wrought?" ran from the Supreme Court chamber in the Capitol in Washington, D.C., back to Mount Clare Station on the first completed telegraph line.

● When you are through at the B&O Railroad Museum, head north on N. Poppleton St. It sits directly across W. Pratt St. from the museum's entrance. The street was named for (and by) an early surveyor, Thomas Poppleton. A map he created in 1822 has his name on this street.

● Just a half block up N. Poppleton St., take a left onto Lemmon St. to visit the Irish Shrine Museum at 918 and 920 Lemmon St. This row of houses was built in 1848 to provide housing for the growing number of workers—most of them Irish—for the B&O Railroad. By the next year, every house on the block was sold; the six-room homes cost $400 each, and everyone who lived here was of Irish descent. Today's Irish Shrine is a unique and little-known museum: one of the houses is decorated in period furnishings, reflecting the immigrant family who lived there in the 1860s. The other house has alternating exhibits related primarily to Irish American life.

● Continuing north on N. Poppleton St., look for St. Peter the Apostle Church at the corner of N. Poppleton St. and Hollins St. This five-columned, Greek Revival building was built in 1842–44 to serve the growing number of Irish newly settled in the area. Baltimore architect Robert Cary Long Jr. designed the church after the Athenian Theseus. Babe Ruth was baptized in this church.

● Continue north on N. Poppleton St. When you reach W. Baltimore St., you'll see two new buildings straddling N. Poppleton that are part of the new University of Maryland BioPark, a real coup for long-neglected West Baltimore. The BioPark is an extension of the University of Maryland, Baltimore, campus and concentrates on biotechnology and community revitalization.

- Continue north on N. Poppleton St. When you reach W. Lexington St., take a left.

- Go a half block and take a right onto N. Amity St. (*Note:* if you are doing this route by car, you will not be able to go north on N. Amity St, as it's one-way. Instead, go one more block to N. Schroeder St.) Just ahead to the right, at 203 N. Amity St., is where Edgar Allan Poe lived with his wife (and cousin), Virginia Clemm; his aunt, Maria Clemm; his grandmother, Elizabeth Cairnes Poe; and his brother, Henry, in the early 1830s. It has been conjectured that in this house Poe wrote and published nine short stories, eight poems, and a slew of reviews. Among these is the oft-anthologized "MS. in a Bottle," for which he won $50 in a contest sponsored by the *Baltimore Saturday Visiter.* It was Poe's first taste of literary success. He also wrote "Berenice," a story about a man obsessed with his ill cousin's teeth, based, Poe said, on the rumors alive in Baltimore at the time that grave robbing was common in the city because dentists were paying top dollar for stolen teeth. Many scholars consider it Poe's first true horror story. There is relatively little of Poe's left in the house (glass-ware, china, a lock of hair, a sextant), but most guests swear to the presence of a particular aura. When the actor Vincent Price visited the house, he is said to have remarked, "This place gives me the creeps." (See "Back Story" on page 116 for changes in the operation of the Poe House.)

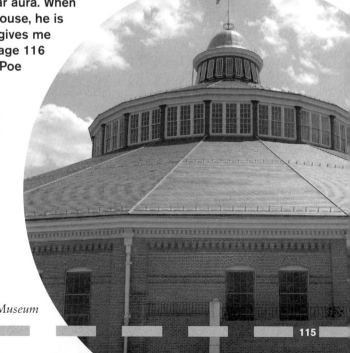

- Return to W. Lexington St. and take a right. Take a left at the next block onto N. Schroeder St., named for a wealthy German family who once owned a Westside Greek Revival mansion.

- Continue on N. Schroeder St. for four blocks and take a right onto Hollins St.

B&O Railroad Museum

Back Story

The Edgar Allan Poe House suffers from its location, literally connected to a public-housing unit and in a neighborhood with no other immediate tourist attractions. As a result, it saw far fewer visitors (roughly 5,000 a year) than its historical and cultural value merit. In 2011, the cash-strapped City of Baltimore decided it could no longer pay for its maintenance. Local fundraisers and general awareness from a wide range of Baltimoreans kept the house operating, but its status as a public museum remained tenuous. (Because it's a historic property, it cannot be torn down. But it did face the danger of the same fate as the Mencken House; see opposite page.) In October 2012, the Poe House closed due to financial constraints. However, and very fortunately, the city agreed to sell it to the B&O Railroad Museum, which will run both properties beginning in spring 2013. It is anticipated that a visitor can buy combination tickets to both museums and enjoy a shuttle between. The arrangement will also result in a tripling of the annual budget to run the Poe House.

● Go one block west on Hollins St. to S. Arlington Ave. and the Hollins Market complex. Originally constructed in 1836–38 and expanded and improved in 1846, 1863–64 (only by Union men; no Confederate-sympathizers need apply), and 1877, the Italianate market is listed on the National Register of Historic Places. While Lexington Market is Baltimore's—and the country's—oldest public market, predating Hollins Market by 110 years, the Hollins Market building is the city's oldest remaining public market building and it anchors the east side of the Union Square–Hollins Market Historic District. Truth is, Hollins lacks the assortment and electricity you find at Lexington Market (and many of the other city markets), but there's still plenty of interest here. Head inside and pick up some food.

Behind the market, at 1115 Hollins St., is the Black Cherry Puppet Theater. (Yes, it really is a puppet theater.)

● Head west on Hollins St. three blocks to S. Calhoun St. The extraordinary building at the corner of Hollins and S. Calhoun is currently home to the Maryland Library

Association. But it began its life as the Enoch Pratt Free Library's No. 2 branch, one of the original four buildings Enoch Pratt bequeathed to Baltimore in 1884 for the creation of the country's first public, urban, free library system. This was H. L. Mencken's local branch and was the laboratory for the Pulitzer Prize–winning author Russell Baker, who grew up nearby. As a child, Baker practically lived in this building, remembering it as "a wonderful, mysterious place with cathedral beams in the ceiling . . . I tried to read my way through the whole place one summer." A similar impulse seized writer Dashiell Hammett, author of *The Maltese Falcon, The Thin Man,* and other famous works, when he lived nearby as a child (at 212 N. Stricker St., since demolished); he once vowed to read every book in the library. It's a striking building with terra-cotta roof panels; quirky chimney designs; and curvy, pitched Romanesque arches.

● Another three blocks west of the Enoch Pratt No. 2 branch building, just beyond S. Stricker St., is Union Square Park (bounded by S. Stricker St., Hollins St., S. Gilmor St., and W. Lombard. St.), a must-see for fans of H. L. Mencken, the "Sage of Baltimore." It's a shame that Mencken isn't better celebrated in Baltimore, as his renown and stature lives on all over the country and world. (Years ago, when my Swiss cousin was in town visiting, his primary and overriding desire was to see where Mencken lived.) At 1524 Hollins St., on the north side of the park, is the H. L. Mencken House, immediately identifiable by the cutout of the irascible, cigar-chomping Mencken peering out at the park through a first-floor window. "It is as much a part of me as my two hands," he wrote of his beloved home. "If I had to leave it I'd be as certainly crippled as if I lost a leg." Mencken lived here for virtually his entire life (1880–1956) and left a literary and cultural legacy that makes him one of the more oft-quoted writers in American history. His 1919 work, *The American Language,* remains an invaluable cultural reference; it was the first studious work that attempted to draw distinctions between British and American English. From this house, Mencken wrote his many columns, edited the works of Theodore Dreiser, and convinced Clarence Darrow to defend John Scopes in the infamous Scopes Monkey Trial (his writings about the small-mindedness involved in that case are classics of American wit). Once a part of the Baltimore City Life Museums, the house is currently—and sadly—closed to the public. However, the Friends of the H. L. Mencken House arrange for visits by appointment. To make an appointment, go to menckenhouse.org.

Mencken enjoyed walking out his front door and spending time in Union Park. Today, bronzed likenesses of Mencken's books ring the fountain in the middle of the park. The 1847 Palladian dome nearby is in desperate need of restoration; hopefully, that is coming soon. The surrounding Union Square neighborhood, glimpsed as you walked along Hollins St. and as you head down S. Stricker (named for John Stricker, the Revolutionary War general and Marylander), dates to 1840. You'll see many Greek Revival, Italianate, and Federal row homes peppered here and there with art galleries and studios.

● Take S. Stricker St. two blocks south to W. Pratt St and take a left.

● Follow W. Pratt St. 10 blocks east back to the B&O Railroad Museum.

POINTS OF INTEREST (START TO FINISH)

B&O Railroad Museum borail.org, 901 W. Pratt St., 410-752-2490

Irish Shrine Museum irishshrine.org, 918 and 920 Lemmon St., 410-669-8154

Edgar Allan Poe House (The Edgar Allan Poe Society of Baltimore) eapoe.org, 203 N. Amity St., 410-396-4883

Hollins Market 26 S. Arlington Ave., 410-685-6169

Black Cherry Puppet Theater info@blackcherry.org, 1115 Hollins St., 410-752-7272

H. L. Mencken House (Friends of the H. L. Mencken House) menckenhouse.org, 1524 Hollins St.

route summary

1. Start at the B&O Railroad Museum.
2. Go north on Poppleton St. to a left on Lemmon St. to the Irish Shrine.
3. Return to Poppleton St. and go north for nine blocks.
4. Turn left onto W. Lexington St.
5. Turn right onto N. Amity St. to the Edgar Allan Poe House.
6. Turn right onto W. Lexington St.
7. Turn left on N. Schroeder St.
8. Turn right onto Hollins St. to Union Square Park.
9. Turn left onto S. Stricker St.
10. Turn left onto W. Pratt St. to the B&O Railroad Museum.

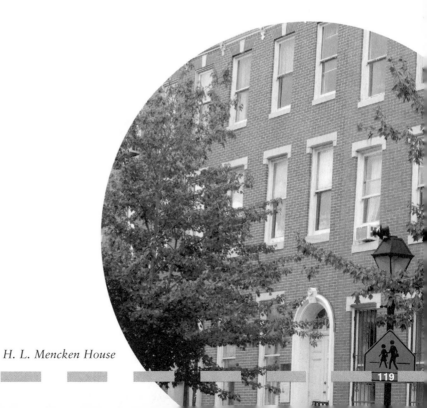

H. L. Mencken House

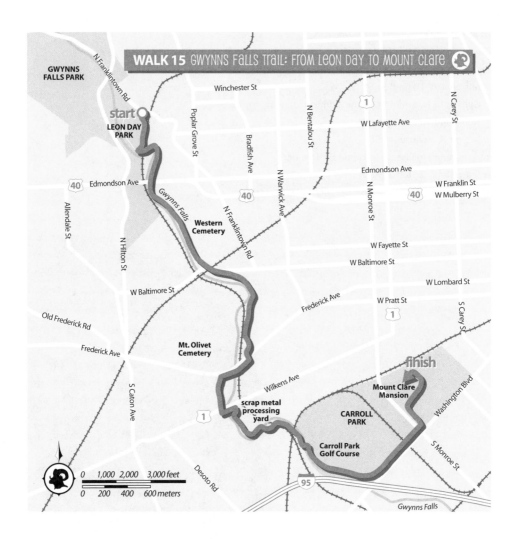

GWYNNS
FALLS PARK

N Franklintown Rd

Winchester St

start
LEON DAY
PARK

Poplar Grove St

Bradfish Ave

N Bentalou St

1

W Lafayette Ave

N Carey St

40 Edmondson Ave

Gwynns Falls

N Warwick Ave

40

N Franklintown Rd

N Monroe St

Edmondson Ave

40

W Franklin St
W Mulberry St

Allendale St

N Hilton St

Western
Cemetery

W Fayette St

W Baltimore St

W Baltimore St

Frederick Ave

W Pratt St
1

W Lombard St

S Carey St

Old Frederick Rd

Frederick Ave

Mt. Olivet
Cemetery

Wilkens Ave

finish

Mount Clare
Mansion

Washington Blvd

S Caton Ave

1

scrap metal
processing
yard

CARROLL
PARK

Carroll Park
Golf Course

S Monroe St

Desoto Rd

95

Gwynns Falls

0   1,000 2,000   3,000 feet

0   200   400   600 meters

15 GWYNNS FALLS Trail:
From LEON Day TO MOUNT CLARE

BOUNDARIES: **N. Franklintown Rd., Washington Blvd.**
DISTANCE: **3.9 miles one way**
DIFFICULTY: **Moderate to strenuous**
PARKING: **At Leon Day Park and on the perimeter of Carroll Park**
PUBLIC TRANSIT: **MTA buses #36 and #51 stop at Carroll Park; MTA bus #35 runs along Wilkens Ave.; MTA bus #10 runs along Frederick Ave.; MTA buses #20 and #30 run along W. Baltimore St.; MTA buses #s 16, 23, 38, and 40 run along Edmondson Ave.**

Captain John Smith, founder of the Jamestown colony in 1607, mapped the Gwynns Falls in 1608, though the Susquehannock and Algonquian Indians had been populating the area for centuries. Smith said the stream tumbled over "felles," or falls, which explains the sometimes confusing local practice of naming streams and rivers "falls" (Jones Falls, Gunpowder Falls). The stream itself was named for Richard Gwynn, who established a trading post here in 1669. The Gwynns Falls, like the Jones Falls, hosted more and more industry over the coming centuries, serving as a natural location for grain mills and slaughterhouses, even while retaining the properties that made it a public recreation spot. In 1904, the famed landscape architects the Olmsted brothers laid out a series of parks and open spaces to be included in their plan for the Greater Baltimore Public Grounds. The modern Gwynns Falls Trail (GFT) resurrects much of that plan. The GFT is a 15-mile greenway snaking its way from and through West Baltimore to the south of the city. The trail has been designated as part of both the East Coast Greenway network of trails from Maine to Florida and the Chesapeake Bay Gateways Network, a system of "parks, refuges, museums, historic sites and water trails spanning the [Chesapeake Bay] watershed." The trail has also become a focal point for city activities, wonderfully packed with hikes, art shows, and cultural festivities of all kinds. The northern reaches of the GFT are covered in this book in Walk 24: Dickeyville & Leakin Park; the southern portions are covered primarily in Walk 2: Gwynns Falls Trail II. This walk takes in the middle portions, running through historic West Baltimore neighborhoods and ending at Mount Clare Mansion, the city's oldest Georgian colonial house.

- Begin at Leon Day Park, which used to be known as the Bloomingdale Oval but was renamed in honor of the West Baltimore resident and baseball all-star who played in the Negro Leagues from 1934 to 1950 and was inducted into the Baseball Hall of Fame in 1995. He spent his playing days with the Baltimore Black Sox and the Baltimore Elite Giants. He grew up in nearby Mt. Winans and returned to live out his days in West Baltimore after his retirement from baseball. The park boasts new facilities, including playgrounds, lighted sports fields, and restrooms. The neighborhood that incorporates Leon Day Park is called Rosemont–Franklintown Road, but before its residential days, in the 1920s and 30s, it was known as Calverton. Then, the area hosted slaughterhouses and five mills, including the Calverton Grain Mill and the Union Abattoir Company. The entire residential neighborhood was almost demolished in the 1960s, when a proposal was put forth to run I-70 through the city. But vociferous opposition halted the plans, and the neighborhood of Rosemont was created. (Thus, one can now see the strange dead end of I-70, which shoots west all the way to Cove Fort, Utah, a couple of miles west, at Trailhead #1 for the GFT.)

- Walk to the end of Leon Day Park and pick up the GFT. You'll be traversing and then paralleling the old Ellicott Driveway, a 19th-century thruway, originally created as a toll pike and today closed to vehicular traffic. The driveway follows the route of a millrace that used to carry water to the Ellicott family's flour-milling complex along the Gwynns Falls. Eventually, some 26 gristmills operated along the falls in the 1800s. But industry had been flourishing there well before that, as companies such as the Baltimore Iron Works were turning out nails and anchors in the early 1700s.

- Follow the GFT as it goes under a steel bridge and parallels the CSX freight tracks and the Gwynns Falls, meandering in the heavily wooded valley to your right. The GFT approaches and then crosses Edmondson Ave. You won't see it in summer, but up the hill to your left is Western Cemetery, more than 250 years old and incorporated in 1846.

- Cross under a bridge and look for the informational sign and benches. The sign will tell you that this section was once known as Baltimore's Niagara Falls, created by the diversion dam for the millrace. You might be tempted to laugh at the hyperbole, but the water pouring over the rocks is really rather nice.

- Emerge from the GFT at W. Baltimore St., and you'll see the beautiful triple-arched Baltimore Street Bridge, constructed in 1932. The GFT parallels W. Baltimore St. to the left for a hundred yards or so, taking you under the bridge and then back into the woods along the Ellicott Driveway.

● The next road up is Frederick Ave. Take a right here, using the road to cross over the CSX tracks and Gwynns Falls (there are GFT signs at all sections where it's not abundantly clear which way to go). Frederick Ave. (MD 144) is still considered a national road, eventually merging with US 40. In the city's earliest days, this road was built as the Baltimore and Frederick Turnpike to connect the city with wheat fields to the west so that products could be transported to the Inner Harbor for shipment. Here, where Frederick Ave. crosses the Gwynns Falls, many mills and other businesses set up shop throughout the 19th century.

● Opposite S. Dukeland St., take a left back into the woods to stay on the GFT. Just a block to the west, bounded to the south by Frederick Rd., is Mt. Olivet Cemetery, the burial place of, among others, figures important to Methodism, including 18th- and 19th-century Bishops Francis Asbury (born in England in 1745 and the first American Methodist bishop), John Emory, Enoch George, and Beverly Waugh, plus Robert Strawbridge, who came to America before its independence and became the country's first Methodist preacher.

● The GFT here passes through some open green space as it approaches Wilkens Ave. There used to be a public, gender-separate swimming pool here, built by the city in the early 20th century when the Gwynns Falls became too polluted for swimming. Wilkens Ave. takes its name from the German immigrant William Wilkens, owner of the nearby Wilkens Curled Hair Factory, which processed animal hair for mattresses and upholstery and operated from 1845 until the

Triple bridges on the Gwynns Falls Trail

1920s. It was Wilkens who set up the city's first telephone line in the 1800s between his factory here and his plant at the Inner Harbor.

- Take a left when you reach Wilkens Ave. and cross over the Gwynns Falls again. Just over the bridge on Wilkens, you'll see the GFT again on the right as it heads back into the woods. Initially, there's a not-too-pleasing scrap-metal processing yard to the left; the area was once the site of the sprawling Union Stockyard, the country's largest stockyard east of Chicago, which operated from 1891 to 1967. But the route becomes quite wooded again, and coming is one of the most interesting and scenic sections of the entire trail: a series of three steel bridges crisscrossing old stone abutments of the former Brunswick Street Bridge. Long before the bridges, American Indians crossed the stream here. A fourth bridge comes soon after, and you'll head under the wagon pass of the old Carrollton Viaduct, the B&O's first bridge, constructed in 1829. The bridge has an impressive 80-foot-diameter center arch (300 feet in total length) and was the country's first stone masonry bridge built for railroading. It remains the world's oldest railway bridge still in use. The viaduct was declared a National Historic Landmark in 1971 and a Historic Civil Engineering Landmark 11 years later.

- The GFT soon skirts the outer edge of Carroll Park Golf Course, one of five city-run golf courses, and emerges at Washington Blvd., becoming—somewhat shockingly after so much green—very urban. Turn left at Washington Blvd., as the GFT parallels the road and soon passes the Montgomery Business Park. This building complex is pretty arresting up close—most area residents know it only from seeing it so prominently from I-95. It's an eight-story, 1.3-million-square-foot complex that has been refurbished in recent years. The Art Deco building once served as the Montgomery Ward Catalog House and Retail Store. When built, in 1925, it was Baltimore's largest mercantile building. It's currently listed on the National Register of Historic Places.

- Continue paralleling Washington Blvd. until you reach S. Monroe St., and cross diagonally to enter Carroll Park. The Carroll family bought 2,500 acres on the Patapsco in 1732, which is today's Carroll Park. Here, Carroll and other business partners formed the Baltimore Iron Works, with its factory upstream along the Gwynns Falls. Aside from many recreational opportunities, the park is most famous for being the home of Mount Clare Mansion, circa 1760, Maryland's first house museum and the oldest colonial Georgian house in Baltimore. There are several paved loops in the park, but to reach the Mount Clare Mansion, head left (north).

Charles Carroll (see "Back Story" in Walk 10 on page 74) began construction on Mount Clare in 1756. The house is a must-see—an absolute beauty of simple, clean Georgian style. And inside, you'll find almost 3,000 original 18th- and 19th-century objects.

● The walk ends here. But there's more of the GFT beyond Carroll Park. Check out the trail map (see "Points of Interest" below). Portions of what lies south of here on the GFT are covered in the following walks: Walk 2: GFT II: Westport Waterfront, Walk 3: Federal Hill, and Walk 4: Inner Harbor Promenade. There's also plenty of public transportation to get you back to Leon Day Park if you don't wish to retrace your steps.

POINTS OF INTEREST (START TO FINISH)

Leon Day Park 1200 block of N. Frankilintown Rd.

Baltimore Street Bridge W. Baltimore St. (between 2500 and 2900 blocks)

Carrollton Viaduct Gwynns Falls, near Carroll Park

Montgomery Park 1800 Washington Blvd.

Mount Clare Museum House, Carroll Park mountclare.org, 1500 Washington Blvd., 410-837-3262

For Gwynns Falls Trail information, visit gwynnsfallstrail.org.

ROUTE SUMMARY

1. Start at Leon Day Park (1200 block of N. Franklintown Rd.).
2. Follow the Gwynns Falls Trail (GFT) across Edmondson Ave. and W. Baltimore St.
3. Turn right onto Frederick Ave.
4. Turn left onto the GFT opposite S. Dukeland St.
5. Turn left onto Wilkens Ave.
6. Turn right onto the GFT.
7. Turn left onto Washington Blvd.
8. Cross S. Monroe St. and enter Carroll Park.

CONNECTING THE WALKS

Taking the GFT in a northeastern direction from Leon Day Park (the opposite direction of this walk) will take you into the heart of Gwynns Falls and Leakin Parks. Access to Walk 24: Dickeyville & Leakin Park is nearby.

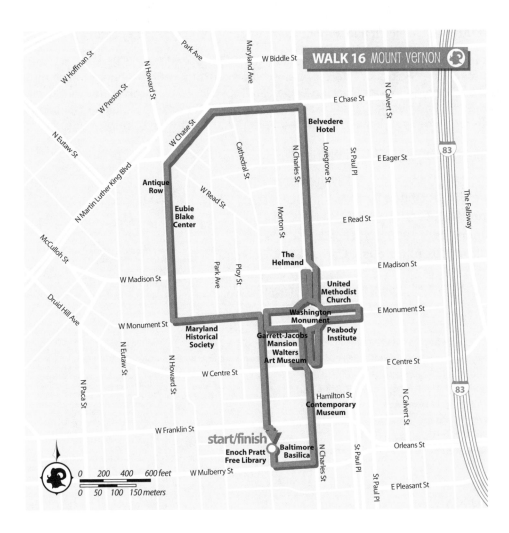

WALK 16 MOUNT VERNON

W Hoffman St

N Howard St

Park Ave

Maryland Ave

W Biddle St

N Calvert St

W Preston St

E Chase St

N Eutaw St

W Chase St

Belvedere Hotel

Cathedral St

N Charles St

Lovegrove St

St Paul Pl

E Eager St

83

N Martin Luther King Blvd

Antique Row

W Read St

Eubie Blake Center

Morton St

E Read St

The Fallsway

McCulloch St

Druid Hill Ave

The Helmand

W Madison St

Park Ave

Ploy St

E Madison St

United Methodist Church

E Monument St

W Monument St

Maryland Historical Society

Washington Monument

Garrett-Jacobs Mansion Walters Art Museum

Peabody Institute

N Eutaw St

N Howard St

W Centre St

E Centre St

N Paca St

Hamilton St

Contemporary Museum

N Calvert St

83

W Franklin St

start/finish

Baltimore Basilica

Orleans St

Enoch Pratt Free Library

N Charles St

St Paul Pl

St Paul Pl

W Mulberry St

E Pleasant St

0   200   400   600 feet
0   50   100   150 meters

16 MOUNT VERNON: BALTIMORE'S DRAWING ROOM

BOUNDARIES: **N. Howard St., W. Mulberry St., St. Paul St., W. Chase St.**
DISTANCE: **2 miles**
DIFFICULTY: **Moderate**
PARKING: **Street parking, with residential restrictions, along route**
PUBLIC TRANSIT: **MTA bus #3 stops at Cathedral and Madison; MTA buses #s 3, 61, 64, and 410 stop at Madison and St. Paul, Centre and St. Paul, Charles and Hamilton, and Charles and Mount Vernon Place; MTA buses #3 and #11 stop at Cathedral and Centre. The free Charm City Circulator Purple bus makes stops in Mount Vernon.**

Today's Mount Vernon, a National Landmark Historic District and a Baltimore City Cultural District, was once part of Revolutionary War hero John Eager Howard's massive estate, Belvidere, a country escape a mile north of Baltimore-Town. As the city grew northward in the early and mid-1800s, it eventually expanded to encompass today's Mount Vernon. Earlier, Howard had donated this chunk of land—the highest in the city—so that it could be graced with the country's first memorial to George Washington. Soon enough, Baltimore's leading citizens and wealthiest families tried to outdo one another in building the fabulous mansions and solid brownstone row homes that give Mount Vernon the beautiful character it still enjoys today; lucky for us, some of these families subsequently tried to outdo one another in their philanthropic activities as well, endowing Baltimore with a treasure trove of cultural institutions. Today's Mount Vernon does what all great urban neighborhoods do: combine history, splendor, entertainment, and an abundance of cultural attractions. On top of all this, it possesses what could easily be the country's most beautiful public square: Mount Vernon Place. The Washington Monument anchors the square, standing sentinel since 1829 (predating D.C.'s more famous monument by 55 years) and surrounded by beautifully landscaped public gardens and fountains and a collection of 19th-century buildings. And that's just one segment of the neighborhood, which radiates from the square and encompasses a bevy of sights and great shops and restaurants. Mount Vernon is Central Baltimore's jewel, a terrific place to wander in awe.

● Start in the 400 block of Cathedral St. On either side of the street, you'll find two wonderful attractions, places for deep contemplation and deep appreciation of architecture, history, and a sense of the spiritually sublime. On the east side of the street is the Baltimore Basilica; on the west side is the central branch of the Enoch Pratt Free Library.

The Baltimore Basilica was the first Catholic cathedral in the New World, built 1806–1821, reflecting Baltimore's status as the first Catholic diocese in the country. Two towering figures in early America oversaw the design and construction of the cathedral: Benjamin Henry Latrobe (the father of American architecture and Thomas Jefferson's Architect of the Capitol) and the country's first bishop, John Carroll (cousin of Charles Carroll, the only Catholic signer of the Declaration of Independence). The Basilica is an important symbol not only for Catholics but also for all Americans in that it represents the flowering of a religious minority in response to the Constitution's newly granted freedom of religion. The architecture was designed to embrace this freedom and to present itself in a truly American style—no more European mimicry. The massive dome, inspired by the U.S. Capitol, lends the building a dramatic flair; many prominent architects consider the Basilica one of the world's finest 19th-century buildings. It is a National Landmark and tours are available. Be sure to check out the basement catacombs, a truly fascinating place.

Across from the Basilica is a place many Baltimoreans find no less spiritual. This story begins in 1882, when wealthy businessman and philanthropist Enoch Pratt offered an endowment of more than a million dollars for the creation of a free library. "My library," Pratt declared, "shall be for all, rich and poor without distinction of race or color, who, when properly accredited, can take out the books if they will handle them carefully and return them." The goal from the start was to have an entire system of branches throughout the city, making it the first public library system in the country. By 1885, the Pratt Library had purchased its first books, and the system's first branch went up in 1886 on nearby Mulberry St. The current building, a grand old beauty, dates to 1931 and has several notable characteristics quite unique in its time: a street-level entrance (as opposed to a grand staircase), as well as the installation of "shop windows" to lure in patrons with the library's offerings. Definitely go inside to see the gorgeous central room with its paintings and skylight, and take the stairs to check out the wonderful smaller rooms and scattered public spaces perfect for curling up with a book—snag a spot in front of a stained glass window, for example. Of particular note are the library's collection of Poe materials and the H. L. Mencken collection, the world's largest, housed in the Mencken reading room.

● Head south on Cathedral St. to your first intersection, W. Mulberry St., and take a left, encircling the Basilica. At the corner, look for the unobtrusive stone marker facing Charles St. This is the George Washington Bicentennial Marker. It dates to 1932 and is one in a series of Washington-Rochambeau Revolutionary Route markers, following the trail of Revolutionary War heroes George Washington and Count Rochambeau. The marker tells you that Count Rochambeau's troops camped here in 1782, when this area was known as Howard's Woods, part of John Eager Howard's estate. The elm tree referred to on the marker is no longer here.

- Go north on N. Charles St. At the end of the block is the Pope John Paul II Prayer Garden; its creation in 2006 raised some controversy, as it involved the regrettable destruction of the beautiful Rochambeau Apartments, built in 1905.

- Cross W. Franklin St., taking note of the striking building on the left, home to the First Unitarian Church of Baltimore, a bastion of liberal Christianity. The church dates to 1817, when a group of Baltimoreans decided to "form a religious society and build a church for Christians who are Unitarian and cherish the liberal sentiments on the subject of religion." By the following year, this domed building was built. A sermon delivered in this church in 1819 essentially defined American Unitarianism. (When Enoch Pratt's first branch on Mulberry was demolished, Pratt donated the used bricks and more money to create the church's parish hall.)

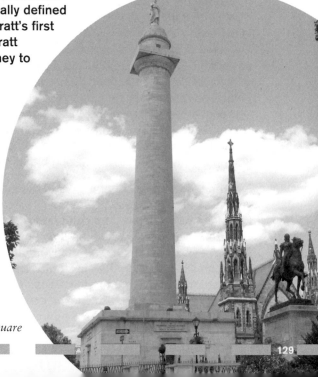

- Continue north on N. Charles St. Just ahead on the right, 505 N. Charles St. was scheduled to be the new home of the Contemporary Museum. However, financial difficulties have forced the museum to suspend operations as of September 2012. The museum's board of directors continues to explore options designed to ensure the Contemporary's return to Baltimore's art scene. Visit contemporary.org for updates.

Washington Monument in Mount Vernon Square

● Head north on N. Charles St. You'll be approaching magnificent Mount Vernon Place, likely among the most gorgeous urban public spaces you'll ever come across. But before you head straight for the incomparable Washington Monument, go left, onto Centre St., and head into the superb Walters Art Museum for more than 35,000 objects on display, ranging more than 55,000 years, from ancient Egyptian, Greek, and Roman to 20th-century European masters. The museum was made possible first through the extraordinary collection (more than 25,000 works of art), and then the generous gift, of William Thompson Walters and his son Henry Walters: the art plus $2 million for maintenance.

The elder Walters made his fortune in railroading and began collecting an amazing array of artworks. After he accumulated wealth, Walters moved his family to the house at 5 W. Mount Vernon Pl. After William's wife died while on a trip to Europe, he began collecting with even more drive. Back in Baltimore, he opened up his house to visitors once a week during the months of April and May so that people could see his collection. He then donated the admission fee to the Baltimore Association for the Improvement in the Condition of the Poor. When William died, son Henry picked up where his father left off, in both business acumen and art collecting. In one amazing acquisition, he purchased the entire contents of a Roman palace containing more than 1,700 pieces. He also possessed his father's charitable streak, first purchasing three adjoining houses on Charles St. and creating a large open space modeled on the University of Genoa's University Palace, and then opening it up to the public to view the art inside. When he died in 1931, he bequeathed the buildings and the collection to the city of Baltimore. (As something of a museum junkie, I never miss an opportunity to visit at the least the principal art museum in any city I visit, in the United States or abroad; invariably, the Walters remains among my favorites for its amazing breadth and sublime setting.)

● Exit the Walters onto Centre St. and take a left, emerging onto N. Charles St. Take your time in this block. The square itself could hold its own against any classic European public plaza. The celebrated 19th-century landscape-architecture firm Carrère & Hastings created the small parks radiating from the monument. The Beaux Arts firm was responsible for many notable buildings and spaces all over the world, including the New York Public Library. Directly opposite the Walters, within a fountain in the middle of curving marble steps, is the beloved Sea Urchin statue, frolicking in a circular pool, what H. L. Mencken called Washington's spittoon. Edward Berge, a prominent Baltimore sculptor who studied under Auguste Rodin, created the urchin statue in 1924. It was originally placed on the Johns Hopkins University Homewood campus; the one you see here is an enlarged reproduction, executed by Edward's son, Henry, in 1961. Behind it, the house at 609 N. Charles, with the double veranda, was once the home of Napoléon Bonaparte's nephew, Jerome.

● You'll feel the pull toward the exquisite Washington Monument, crowned with its namesake hero, arm outstretched and pointing south toward the harbor. Promotional material will consistently trumpet the notion that this is the country's first monument to Washington. In fact, that's not technically true. The country's first and thus oldest monument to George Washington (1827) is in Washington Monument State Park in Boonsboro, Western Maryland, but the monument that towers over Mt. Vernon Square in Baltimore is older than D.C.'s more famous cousin and is infinitely more attractive. For more on the monument, see "Back Story" on page 134. For now, head inside and climb the 228 steps to check out a terrific view of the city. Also inside you'll find a bust of Washington, created by the 18th-century Italian sculptor Giuseppe Ceracchi in 1791–92.

The monument also serves as the center point to so many Mount Vernon traditions. During First Thursday activities, from May through October, free concerts take place here. Flower Mart has been held every May for more than 100 years; it's a wonderful festival featuring hundreds of vendors associated with flowers and gardening. Every September, you'll find the Baltimore Book Festival, an annual attraction that regularly draws more than 50,000 visitors over the three-day weekend and is the largest festival of its kind in the country. And, of course, there's the annual Monument Lighting in December, when old George gets decked in lights and washed in fireworks to usher in the holiday season.

● Standing in front of the monument to Washington is the fine sculpture to the Marquis de Lafayette, the valiant Frenchman who served under George Washington in the Continental Army and who became an American hero. When Lafayette visited the United States in 1825, as a guest of President James Monroe, he created a sensation everywhere he went, and he went to a lot of places, visiting all 24 states and logging some 6,000 miles. He was given honorary American citizenship and when he died he was buried in France with American soil from Bunker Hill. This bronze, depicting the heroic and serene Lafayette atop a straining, muscular horse, was dedicated in 1924. President Calvin Coolidge was on hand for the dedication.

● With the monuments to Washington and Lafayette in front of you, head left, down W. Mount Vernon Pl. In his 1905 book, *The American Scene,* author Henry James wrote of this block, "I felt quite as the visitor as yet unintroduced may feel during some long preliminary wait in a drawing-room." The glorious house on the corner is the Hackerman House, built 1859–61 (the square's second-oldest house) and formerly the Thomas-Jencks-Gladding Mansion. The Thomas in the name was John, the original owner; he was a descendent of John Hanson, the president of the Congress under the Articles of Confederation. The next owners hosted high-society parties inside, enjoying a guest list that reached into the upper echelons of society, such as President Warren Harding and President Herbert Hoover's wife, Lou Henry. Willard and Lillian Hackerman donated the house to the city in 1984; it became Walters's property the following year and today it houses the museum's Asian-art collection.

● Continue down the hill; three more house fronts to the left is the magnificent Garrett-Jacobs Mansion. This extraordinary manse combined the work of two of America's most influential architects: John Russell Pope and Stanford White. John W. Garrett, president of the B&O Railroad, originally bought the house at 11 W. Mount Vernon Pl. in 1872 as a wedding gift for his son and daughter-in-law. It was the architect White who created this house, as well as the addition of #9, which he joined to #11. Mr. Garrett's widow, remarried to Dr. Henry Barton Jacobs, purchased #7 and had John Russell Pope design the new addition. All these additions (including the rear of #13) made it, by some accounts, the second-largest private home in the United States after the White House: some 40 rooms, 100 windows, and 16 fireplaces. There was an art gallery, a theater, a conservatory, a dining room with musicians' balcony, and an elevator. It was the scene of some of the finest hostessing anywhere in the country. The Jacobs lived there into the 1930s; the Engineering Society of Baltimore (the Engineers Club) bought the house in 1962 and has continued as owner, restoring the house to much of its original grandeur. Tours of the house can be arranged; see "Points of Interest" on page 138.

● When you reach the end of the block, Cathedral St., go right, staying in Mount Vernon Place. At the intersection of W. Mount Vernon Pl. and Cathedral St. is the Renaissance Revival Severn apartment building, designed in 1885 by Baltimore architect Charles E. Cassell. While homes like the Garrett-Jacobs Mansion get a lot of attention, and rightly so, check out the other houses that line the square—no slouches here. Near Cathedral St., you'll see another gift of William Walters, a replica of Paul Dubois's *Military Courage* statue, installed in 1885. *Courage* is one of four statues (the others are Faith, Meditation, and Charity) that serve as pillars at the tomb of General Jucault de Lamoricière, a commander of the French army in North Africa, in Nantes Cathedral, France.

The oldest house on the square is 8 W. Mount Vernon Pl. It was built in 1842 and was known originally as the Tiffany-Fisher House, owned by William Tiffany. It's a Greek Revival home, as evidenced by the Doric columns over the entranceway. Today, and since 1942, it is home to the Mount Vernon Club, an elite private women's social club. Local Wallis Warfield, when she became the Duchess of Windsor after the former King Edward VIII abdicated his throne to marry her, stayed here with her royal beau in 1959. (Warfield was named for her uncle, Severn Teackle Wallis, whose bronzed likeness is nearby—see page 135.)

As you head back toward the Washington Monument, you'll see in the green median to your right a bronze lion. The lion also once belonged to William Walters. It is the work of noted French sculptor Antoine-Louis Barye. This is also a replica; the original can be found in the Tuileries in Paris.

● Take a left when you reach the cobblestone circle onto N. Washington Pl. You'll immediately see the gorgeous Washington Apartments at #700. This building was constructed in 1906 in a terrific Beaux Arts style. Next to the apartment building is the Stafford, originally a hotel built in 1894 and now an apartment building for students at Johns Hopkins. F. Scott Fitzgerald, among other notables, resided for a time here. Charles E. Cassell designed this building too, the tallest on the square when it was built, as well as the house next door, the French château-style Graham-Hughes House (1895).

To your right is another bronze, this one to local hero John Eager Howard, dedicated in 1904. It's fitting Howard should be here, as this land was once part of his sprawling estate. His desire for a Washington monument was derived primarily from his having served directly under General George in the Continental Army. The two small circles on the back of the statue's base depict the medal Howard received from Congress for his valor at the Battle of Cowpens, as well as a panel depicting a Continental officer (presumably Howard) harassing a British soldier.

Behind Howard, occupying a sunny spot facing the Washington Monument, is the bronze likeness of Roger Brooke Taney, a Marylander and the fifth Chief Justice of the Supreme Court. Taney has the ignominious distinction of authoring the famous

Back Story

In 1809, 10 years after George Washington died, Baltimore citizens petitioned the Maryland General Assembly to raise money to honor the nation's first president. It took 20 years to complete, making the simple circular cairn in Boonsboro older by two years. Because the cornerstone was laid in 1815, many people consider the monument the country's first. The site originally chosen for the monument was at Calvert and Fayette, where the War Memorial stands today (see Walk 12: Downtown: Contrasts), but area residents feared the potential of a falling column. John Eager Howard came to the rescue again, donating the land where Washington stands today.

Washington is 16 feet high and weighs 30 tons, made of marble mined in Baltimore County. One of the monument's more memorable descriptions comes from a fictional character, Herman Melville's Ishmael, who in the chapter "The Mast-Head" in *Moby Dick* remarks, "Great Washington . . . stands high aloft on his towering main-mast in Baltimore, and like one of Hercules' pillars, his column marks that point of human grandeur beyond which few mortals will go." The stately general is depicted in Roman toga handing over his commission as commander in chief. Appropriately, he faces the statehouse in Annapolis, where in real life he performed that act—sans toga.

Dred Scott decision, which held that slaves escaping to freedom had no rights as Americans. Taney even went so far as to claim that no people of African descent or their descendents, whether they were slaves or not, were citizens of the United States and thus were not protected by the Constitution. That decision, upheld by the court 7-2 but later deemed a blatant misreading of the law, is forever linked with Taney. When Taney died, President Abraham Lincoln did not acknowledge him. In 1865, Congress rejected a proposal to create a bust of Taney to be displayed along with the four Chief Justices who preceded him. But he was a man of legal distinction despite the controversy. He had served as Maryland's Attorney General as well as the country's 12th Attorney General and had practiced law in Frederick with his partner Francis Scott Key. He died on the very day Maryland officially abolished slavery. The bronze you see is a recast of the 1871 sculpture that stands outside the Maryland statehouse in Annapolis (a frequent target of protests by Marylanders wishing him to be taken away from this prominent spot). This, too, was a gift of the Walters family.

To Taney's left is the stunning Mount Vernon Place United Methodist Church, a Victorian Gothic beauty, completed in 1872 and designed to serve as a Methodist "cathedral." Its most striking aspect is the color, a greenish tint that comes from the stone used to construct it: green serpentine marble from the Bare Hills section of Baltimore County, just over the city line near Falls Rd. The church's original organ ran on water power and was, at the time, the fourth-largest organ in the country. Today, the church uses a magnificent M.P. Moller organ, which has almost 3,300 pipes. If you look to the left of the entrance doors, you'll see a plaque telling you that Francis Scott Key died on this spot in 1843 when Charles Howard's mansion stood here. Howard was the son of John Eager Howard and was married to Key's daughter Elizabeth. Key was buried in Old Saint Paul's Cemetery, a couple of miles away, for the next 23 years, but his body was moved in 1866 to his family's ancestral home, Terra Rubra in Carroll County, Maryland.

Next door to the church, at 10 E. Mount Vernon Pl. (left from the Washington Monument) is the Italianate Renaissance Asbury House (1855), named for the first bishop of the Methodist Church in America, Francis Asbury, who preached in Baltimore. The church uses the home as offices and a parish.

● Continue around the block by heading down the hill on E. Mt. Vernon Pl., passing gorgeous brownstones between #22 and #32, a section known as Brownstone Row, built during the Civil War, until you soon reach St. Paul St. (It's probably worth a quick detour to head down E. Monument St. one block to a left onto Calvert St., where you'll see Center Stage on the left. A true success story for smaller regional professional theater, Center Stage, Maryland's state theater, has been putting on terrific shows at reasonable prices since 1963.) Stay in the park area by heading right at St. Paul, passing the monument to Severn Teackle Wallis. Wallis was a famous lawyer in his time (1816–1894); he stands here looking very serious and urbane, his left hand crooked to his midsection, his right atop a pile of papers. Wallis served in the Maryland Legislature and was one of the leaders opposing the Civil War. That opposition landed him in federal prisons, though he was never charged with any crime. He was also a celebrated writer, penning many works, including his most beloved, *Glimpses of Spain* and *Discourse on the Life and Character of George Peabody*. Today, he's buried in Greenmount Cemetery (see Walk 21: Station North). Teackle Alley is located in Mount Vernon, a few blocks away.

Behind Wallis is the lovely Naiad sculpture, constantly sprayed by water, gracefully arched back, by renowned Baltimore sculptor Grace Turnbull.

● Stay on the square by heading right at the end of the block, E. Mount Vernon Pl. Just up the hill on your left is the Baltimore institution associated with the philanthropist George Peabody. At 1 E. Mount Vernon Pl. is the Peabody Institute of the Johns Hopkins University. The Institute is the second-oldest continuously operating conservatory in the country and is today recognized as one of the world's foremost training centers for musicians. The list of prominent faculty and alumni associated with the Peabody is extremely impressive. Peabody was a merchant who made a fortune in dry goods. After moving to London and making a further fortune as a financier, Peabody endowed his old hometown with $1.4 million to create a cultural institution. As he wrote to several friends, "I have determined . . . to establish and endow an Institute in this city, which I hope may become useful towards the improvement of the moral and intellectual culture of the inhabitants of Baltimore, and collaterally to those of the State; and also, towards the enlargement and diffusion of a taste for the Fine Arts." The building you see dates to the 1850s and is in the Renaissance Revival style. To the right of the main entrance are a concert hall, classrooms, an art gallery, and the Peabody Conservatory. On the east side of the building, at 17 E. Mount Vernon, is the magnificent Peabody Library (1875–78), simply one of the finest public rooms anywhere. The Peabody Library is of neo-Greco design and contains six levels of books, soaring more than 60 feet to an open skylight with decorative pillars as supports. Cast-iron balconies face each level and allow you to look down upon the marble floor and get close to that beautiful skylight. There are more than 300,000 volumes in the collection, mostly dating from the 18th and 19th centuries. Definitely head inside to see this wondrous space.

Directly across from the Peabody buildings, in the park median, sits Peabody himself in bronze, facing the Washington Monument.

● When you get to the end of the block, take a right onto N. Charles St., passing the Washington Monument on your left and leaving Mt. Vernon Square. As soon as you leave, you'll see plenty of shops, galleries, and restaurants. Just to the left is a local favorite, The Helmand, a restaurant offering authentic Afghani food run by the family of Afghanistan President Hamid Karzai. In all, there are close to 50 restaurants in Mount Vernon; for a comprehensive list, check out mvcd.org/restaurants. In addition to The Helmand, local favorites include Tio Pepe, The Brewer's Art, Sammy's Trattoria, Ixia, and Mick O'Shea's.

● There's plenty of interesting and attractive architecture as you head north on Charles St. But undoubtedly your eye will be drawn to the looming Beaux Arts masterpiece, the Belvedere, just before Chase St., which you'll reach in four blocks from Mount Vernon Square. A half century of Mount Vernon's prominence had already elapsed when the Belvedere was constructed in 1903, taking its name from the same name (slightly different spelling) of John Eager Howard's estate. It was designed from the start to attract the city's elites; today it houses condos.

❶ Head inside; in the lobby you'll see framed photographs of the Belvedere's many celebrity visitors from its 110 years of existence. Make sure also to head to the left and visit the Owl Bar, one of the city's great bars. It was a hit from the day it opened its doors, attracting locals and travelers passing through. During Prohibition, it operated as a speakeasy and it continues today as a wonderful old place, full of charm and character and darn good cocktails. If it's early in the day, don't sweat it; it's five o'clock somewhere in the world.

● At Chase St., take a left and follow it as it curves around and then take a left onto N. Howard St. You'll be entering the 800 block of N. Howard, a stretch known as Antique Row. There's little question that Antique Row has, unfortunately, lost much of its past splendor, but there are still some shops holding on here and if you're in the market for some antiques, there's a decent chance you can still find what you're looking for. If nothing else, it's worth strolling this block because of its historic association, as this is the oldest antiques district in the country, dating from the 1840s.

● Continue to 847 N. Howard to visit the Eubie Blake National Jazz Institute and Cultural Center, a tribute to the great African American composer and Baltimorean Eubie Blake. Born in the 1880s to parents who had been slaves, he lived for almost a century (there is some discrepancy about his actual birth year). His most famous composition was "I'm Just Wild About Harry," and a young Josephine Baker got her start in one of his shows. The "Institute" in his name focuses on bringing "creative expression and urban consciousness to Baltimore through visual and performing arts education and development opportunities for children, youth and adults in our community." The Institute includes a museum, gallery, gift shop, and studios.

● Two blocks away is W. Monument St., where you should take a left and proceed to #201, where you'll find the Maryland Historical Society, a not-to-be-missed institution fascinating for Marylanders and non-Marylanders alike. Dating to 1844, the MdHS is the state's oldest continuously operating cultural institution. It has been operating out of this building, the former home of Enoch Pratt, since 1919. The Society's collection includes more than 350,000 objects and a library with an astounding seven million books and documents. The museum's collection includes one of only three surviving Revolutionary War officers' uniforms in America, a plethora of colonial artifacts (including the papers of state first families Lords Baltimore and Carroll), and many American Indian pieces predating the country. But without question, the largest attraction by far is the original manuscript of Francis Scott Key's "Star-Spangled Banner." In addition to this sacred piece of Americana, the museum tells the long and unique story of Maryland and the lives of Marylanders and the influence this small state, once dubbed "America in Miniature" by *National Geographic* founder Gilbert Grosvenor, has had on the rest of the country from its inception to today. Because you just came from the Eubie Blake center on Howard St., be sure also to check out the Society's extensive collection of Blake memorabilia.

● Straight ahead on W. Monument you'll see Mount Vernon Square, where you can end your walk. If you wish to end up where you began, however, take the first right just before the square, onto Cathedral St., and the Basilica and Enoch Pratt Central Branch will be three and a half blocks to the south.

POINTS OF INTEREST (START TO FINISH)

The Baltimore Basilica baltimorebasilica.org, 409 Cathedral St., 410-727-3565

Enoch Pratt Free Library, Central Branch prattlibrary.org, 400 Cathedral St., 410-396-5430

First Unitarian Church of Baltimore 12 W. Franklin St., 410-685-2330

The Contemporary Museum contemporary.org

The Walters Art Museum thewalters.org, 600 N. Charles St., 410-547-9000

Washington Monument and Museum at Mount Vernon Place 699 N. Charles St., 410-396-1049

Garrett-Jacobs Mansion/Engineers Club garrettjacobsmansion.org, 11 W. Mount Vernon Pl., 410-539-6914

Mount Vernon Place United Methodist Church mvp-umc.org, 10 E. Mount Vernon Pl.

Peabody Institute of The Johns Hopkins University peabody.jhu.edu, 1 E. Mount Vernon Pl., 410-234-4500

Peabody Library peabodyevents.library.jhu.edu, 17 E. Mount Vernon Pl., 410-234-4943

The Helmand helmand.com, 806 N. Charles St., 410-752-0311

Owl Bar at the Belvedere theowlbar.com, 1 E. Chase St., 410-347-0888

Eubie Blake National Jazz Institute and Cultural Center eubieblake.org, 847 N. Howard St., 410-225-3130

Maryland Historical Society mdhs.org, 201 W. Monument St., 410-685-3750

route summary

1. Start at the 400 block of N. Cathedral St.
2. Turn left onto W. Mulberry St.
3. Turn left onto N. Charles St.
4. Turn left down W. Mount Vernon Pl.
5. Turn right at Cathedral St.
6. Turn right down W. Mount Vernon Pl.
7. Turn left down Washington Pl.
8. Turn right at Madison St.
9. Turn right down Washington Pl.
10. Turn left onto E. Mount Vernon Pl.
11. Turn right at St. Paul St.
12. Turn right down E. Mount Vernon Pl.
13. Turn right down N. Charles St.
14. Go north on Washington Pl./N. Charles St.
15. Turn left onto W. Chase St.
16. Turn left onto N. Howard St.
17. Turn left onto W. Monument St.

connecting the walks

When you took a left onto W. Chase St. from N. Charles, you can go one more block north, to Biddle St., which intersects with Walk 20: Mount Royal.

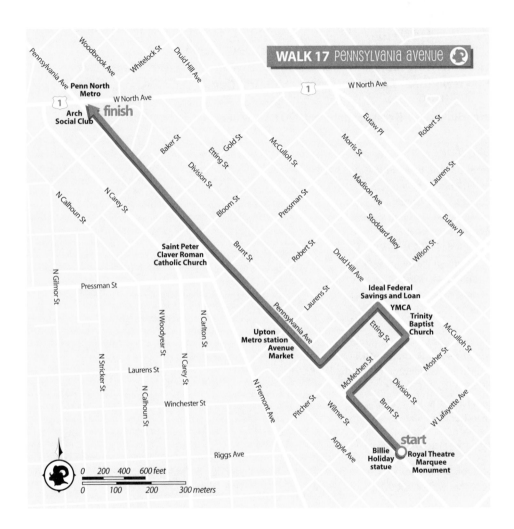

WALK 17 Pennsylvania Avenue

Pennsylvania Ave
Woodbrook Ave
Whitelock St
Druid Hill Ave
W North Ave
Penn North Metro
W North Ave
Arch Social Club
finish
Eutaw Pl
Robert St
Morris St
Baker St
Gold St
McCulloh St
Madison Ave
Laurens St
Etting St
Division St
Pressman St
Bloom St
Stoddard Alley
Eutaw Pl
N Carey St
Wilson St
N Calhoun St
Brunt St
Robert St
Saint Peter Claver Roman Catholic Church
Druid Hill Ave
Ideal Federal Savings and Loan
N Gilmor St
Pressman St
Laurens St
YMCA
Trinity Baptist Church
Etting St
McCulloh St
N Woodyear St
N Carlton St
Pennsylvania Ave
Upton Metro station Avenue Market
McMechen St
Mosher St
N Stricker St
N Carey St
Laurens St
Division St
W Lafayette Ave
N Calhoun St
Winchester St
N Fremont Ave
Pitcher St
Wilmer St
Brunt St
start
Royal Theatre Marquee Monument
Riggs Ave
Argyle Ave
Billie Holiday statue

0 200 400 600 feet
0 100 200 300 meters

17 Pennsylvania Avenue: Harlem Renaissance South

BOUNDARIES: **Pennsylvania Ave., McMechen St., Druid Hill Ave., Wilson St.**
DISTANCE: **1.1 mile**
DIFFICULTY: **Easy**
PARKING: **Street parking, with some restrictions, along route**
PUBLIC TRANSIT: **Upton Metro stop, Penn/North Metro stop, MTA bus #7 runs up and down Pennsylvania Ave.**

To have been here in the early to mid-20th century! Unfortunately, much of Pennsylvania Avenue's glorious past has disappeared under urban ills. Today, the incredible cultural history that took place here is tough to spot—but not impossible. At one time, Pennsylvania Avenue was African American Baltimore's cultural mecca, supporting half a dozen flourishing clubs and hosting the biggest names in entertainment of the day, names that resonate through the decades. The sheer number of African American luminaries to shine in clubs up and down Pennsylvania Avenue made it one of the premier arts destinations in the United States. And in a deeply segregated town, one of the wonderful by-products of so much creativity was a mixed crowd of patrons breaking the social taboos of the time in search of great entertainment. The city's black elite congregated here, and Pennsylvania Avenue was home to many lawyers and doctors. The area also birthed and hosted many important figures of the civil rights movement. It takes a bit of squinting to see it now, but this under-heralded stretch of the Westside deserves a new look. *Note:* much of the information herein comes from the Pennsylvania Avenue Heritage Trail website: pennsylvaniaavenuebaltimore.com.

● Begin at the corner of Pennsylvania Ave. and W. Lafayette Ave. Sitting catty-corner from one another across Pennsylvania Ave. are two attractions. On the east side of the street is the Royal Theatre Marquee Monument. It's a rather poignant site: the marquee stands, looking somewhat neglected, not far from where the old majestic theater once stood. The Royal was demolished in 1971, a sad and undeserved fate for such an institution. Opened in 1922 as the Douglass Theatre, it was one of five theaters, including the famous Apollo in Harlem, designed for black performers to make the rounds. The list of African American stars who have played at the Royal is incredible: Louis

Armstrong, Charlie Parker, Fats Waller, Nat King Cole, The Supremes, Count Basie, Louis Jordan, Duke Ellington, James Brown, Stevie Wonder, The Temptations, Solomon Burke, The Platters, Patti LaBelle, Jackie Wilson, and many others. Both Pearl Bailey and Ethel Waters made their debuts at the Royal, and the legendary boxer Jack Johnson fought an exhibition match here. Comics also played the Royal, including Redd Foxx, Slappy White, and Moms Mabley.

● Across Pennsylvania Ave. and W. Lafayette Ave. is a statue of Billie Holiday. Though not a native, she spent her formative, and very difficult, early years here (see "Back Story" on page 144). Her return to Baltimore as an adult was triumphant: she headlined at the Royal and the Club Tijuana and played legendary shows at the Club Astoria. Holiday wasn't the only Baltimorean to play the Avenue clubs. Eubie Blake, Chick Webb, and Cab Calloway also worked Pennsylvania Avenue, mere blocks from where they were born and raised.

● Continue northwest along Pennsylvania Ave. #1528 was the site of The Comedy Club, run by jazz great Ike Dixon. Duke Ellington remembered Dixon's band, Ike Dixon and the Jazz Demons, as the best band in the city. Dixon's Comedy Club hosted many of the greats, including Miles Davis and Dinah Washington. His hotel above the club provided beds for many touring musicians who would gather to play, chat, and sack out after their shows up and down the block. The club closed in 1964.

● At McMechen St., take a right. Follow McMechen St. past Division St. to Druid Hill Ave.

● Take a left on Druid Hill Ave. There, across the street, you will see Trinity Baptist Church. Founded in 1888, the church is notable primarily because its founder, the Reverend Dr. Gamett Russell Waller, cofounded the Baltimore chapter of the NAACP and was an early member of W. E. B. Dubois's Niagara Movement, a forerunner to the NAACP.

● Next to Trinity, at 1609 Druid Hill Ave., is the YMCA. The Colored Branch of the YMCA was inaugurated in Baltimore in 1885, with Frederick Douglass headlining. It would be another quarter century before the YMCA would have a permanent home, which is what you see in front of you.

● At the corner, at 1629 Druid Hill Ave., is the Ideal Federal Savings and Loan. It looks unassuming, but it has a large role in the financial history of Baltimore and in

Maryland. Begun in 1920, it is the oldest continuously operating African American financial institution in the state.

- You might notice that the next cross street—Wilson St.—is labeled Islamic Way. That's because at 514 Wilson St., just to the left, is the Baltimore Masjid, the city's oldest Islamic place of worship. Baltimore's Islamic community was formed in 1943 and moved to this facility at 514 Wilson St./Islamic Way in 1959. The building itself was constructed in 1880, when it functioned as a livery stable.

- Continue on Wilson St./Islamic Way to the next cross street, Division St. Two houses to the left, #1632, is the childhood home of Thurgood Marshall, the nation's first African American Supreme Court Justice, as the plaque on the side of the brick house with the semicircular entrance will tell you. Not surprisingly, considering the deep racial prejudices of the time, Marshall wasn't terribly fond of his hometown. (See "Back Story" on page 144.)

- Continue on Wilson St. and you'll soon reach Pennsylvania Ave. again. Take a right.

A series of paintings honoring some of the stars who played here, including Cab Calloway, Duke Ellington, Miles Davis, Baltimore School for the Arts graduate Tupac Shakur, James Brown, Ella Fitzgerald, and others, can be found three storefronts to the right. Two storefronts to the left is a wonderful black-and-white mural depicting major figures in African American history, including two Marylanders: Harriet Tubman and Frederick Douglass. Across the street from that mural is Avenue Market, originally established in 1871. Pop in today to pick up some terrific soul food.

Billie Holiday statue

Back Story

Many sources state that Billie Holiday was born in Baltimore, but in fact, she was born in Philadelphia. Her mother brought her to Baltimore as an infant to live with relatives. Here, she endured a rough childhood: often separated from her mother, witness to prostitution, raped, the city did not serve her well. By the time she was a teenager, she had gone to New York, where she would soon begin a remarkable career that left her voice one of the signature sounds of the 20th century.

Maryland has also had a somewhat difficult relationship with its native son, Thurgood Marshall. State officials renamed Baltimore-Washington International Airport the Thurgood Marshall BWI Airport in 2005 and the University of Maryland's Law Library is the Thurgood Marshall Law Library. There's understandable pride in being able to claim the nation's first African American Supreme Court Justice, but his distaste for the segregated city and state of his youth is well documented. Indeed, it was the University of Maryland's refusal to accept him based on his race in 1930 that cemented his drive to fight for legal integration.

- Just up Pennsylvania Ave. to the left, before Laurens St., is the Upton Metro station. Duck inside to see the wonderful Romare Bearden mosaic mural, *Baltimore Uproar,* featuring Billie Holiday leading half a dozen musicians in song. Bearden created the mosaic in 1982, six years before he died. Keep your eye out for two more wonderful murals up ahead on Pennsylvania.

- Across N. Fremont Ave., to the left, is the Saint Peter Claver Roman Catholic Church, a unique institution. Saint Peter Claver was known as the apostle to the slaves, and this is the world's first church dedicated to him. The church, founded in 1888, runs a school that remains the state's oldest African American private school. Many church members played prominent roles during the civil rights era.

- At 2115 Pennsylvania Ave., you'll have to use your imagination. It's a difficult task envisioning what was once here: The Sphinx Club. It was one of the first minority-owned businesses in the country and had, in its heyday, earned an air of exclusivity.

The club actually hasn't been gone that long; after a half-century run, it managed to stay in business until the mid-1990s, making it the area's last major club in existence.

● Last up is the Arch Social Club, at 2426 Pennsylvania Ave. The club remains a vital part of the community, as it has for the last 100 years. Though founded in 1912, the club's current location dates only to 1972. The upper portion of the building that houses the club is much older and retains some of its faded glory; it's architecturally beautiful despite the peeling paint and hints of neglect. From the start, the club's main mission was to promote and support community activities and build stronger neighborhoods. The club's band was led by John Kier, of the Duke Ellington Orchestra.

● The walk ends here, at the intersection of Pennsylvania Ave. and North Ave. The Penn North Metro stop is at the corner and you can use it to get to your next destination.

POINTS OF INTEREST (START TO FINISH)

Royal Theatre Marquee Monument Pennsylvania Ave. and W. Lafayette Ave.

Billie Holiday Plaza 1386 Pennsylvania Ave. at W. Lafayette Ave.

Trinity Baptist Church 1600 Druid Hill Ave.

YMCA 1609 Druid Hill Ave.

Ideal Federal Savings and Loan 1629 Druid Hill Ave.

Baltimore Masjid 514 Islamic Way

Thurgood Marshall Childhood Home 1632 Division St.

Avenue Market 1700 Pennsylvania Ave.

Romare Bearden Mural Upton Metro Station, Pennsylvania Ave.

Saint Peter Claver Roman Catholic Church 1546 N. Fremont Ave.

ROUTE SUMMARY

1. Start at the corner of Pennsylvania Ave. and W. Lafayette Ave.
2. Go northwest on Pennsylvania Ave.
3. Turn right on McMechen St.
4. Turn left on Druid Hill Ave.
5. Turn left on Wilson St./Islamic Way.
6. Turn right on Pennsylvania Ave.

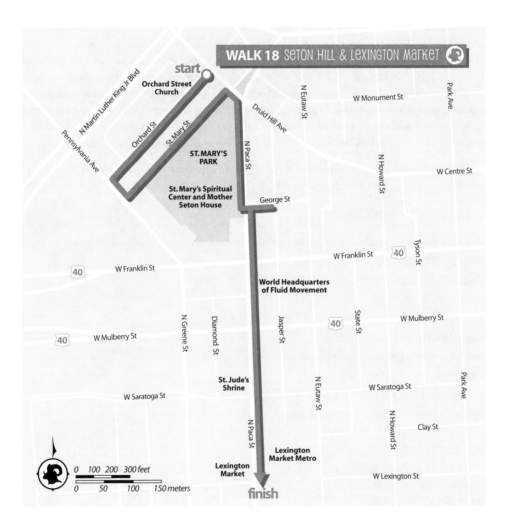

WALK 18 Seton Hill & Lexington Market

start

Orchard Street Church

Orchard St

St. Mary St

N Martin Luther King Jr Blvd

Pennsylvania Ave

ST. MARY'S PARK

St. Mary's Spiritual Center and Mother Seton House

N Paca St

Druid Hill Ave

N Eutaw St

W Monument St

Park Ave

N Howard St

W Centre St

George St

W Franklin St

W Franklin St

40

Tyson St

World Headquarters of Fluid Movement

40

N Greene St

Diamond St

Jasper St

40

State St

W Mulberry St

40

W Mulberry St

W Mulberry St

St. Jude's Shrine

N Eutaw St

W Saratoga St

Park Ave

W Saratoga St

N Paca St

N Howard St

Clay St

Lexington Market Metro

Lexington Market

W Lexington St

finish

0   100 200 300 feet
0   50   100 150 meters

18 SETON HILL & LEXINGTON MARKET: SAINTS AND THE REST OF US

BOUNDARIES: **Druid Hill Ave., Orchard St., N. Paca St.**
DISTANCE: **1.3 miles**
DIFFICULTY: **Easy**
PARKING: **Street parking on Druid Hill Ave. and Orchard St.**
PUBLIC TRANSIT: **Lexington Market has both subway and Light Rail stops, as well as numerous bus-line stops: MTA buses #s 5, 15, 19, 23, and 27. MTA bus #5 stops at Druid Hill Ave. and Orchard St.**

Seton Hill is easy to miss; because it sits in a pocket to the southeast of the major Martin Luther King Jr. Blvd. and is bracketed by busy streets all around (US 40, Pennsylvania Ave., Druid Hill Ave., N. Paca St., and N. Eutaw St.), most people speed by without knowing much about the extraordinary history just down the side streets. Seton Hill dates to the 18th century and was once known as the city's French Quarter for serving as the home of the Parisian priests of the Order of St. Sulpice. This short walk takes in the little enclave's major historical points, full of American firsts: first Catholic seminary, home of the first American-born Catholic saint, first free school for girls, first neo-Gothic architecture. Seton Hill is also home to a historic church that once served as a stop on the Underground Railroad and barely survived the wrecker's ball. And nearby is the country's longest continuously operating market, dating back to 1782. Additionally, Seton Hill showcases some of Baltimore's oldest intact row homes. It's little wonder that the entire neighborhood has been listed on the National Register of Historic Places.

● If driving, park anywhere near Druid Hill Ave. and Orchard St. You're in the heart of Seton Hill and the history comes at you immediately. The street itself recalls the late-18th-century fruit orchard that stood on the spot. At 512 Orchard St. stands the Orchard Street Church, now home to the Baltimore Urban League. Truman Pratt—who had once been a slave belonging to John Eager Howard, the prominent Maryland politician and soldier—founded the church in 1825. The current Italianate structure dates from 1882. Evidence exists that the church site was once part of the Underground Railroad.

- Continue down Orchard St. You will soon pass Tessier St. to the left; the name has significance. Tessier is Father Jean Marie Tessier, one of the Parisian priests of the Order of St. Sulpice. In 1791, Tessier and others came to Baltimore from France and founded St. Mary's Seminary, the first Catholic seminary in the United States. Much of St. Mary's still exists, in pristine condition, and you'll be headed there next.

- When you reach Pennsylvania Ave., turn left. If you had continued down Pennsylvania Ave. to Franklin St. (US 40), you'd be standing where the original town of One Mile Tavern stood in 1791, when the Sulpician priests opened a headquarters to establish their order. You'd have a hard time imagining what the area looked like some 220 years ago, so instead of walking to that not terribly attractive corner, turn left on St. Mary St.

- Almost immediately, you'll be paralleling St. Mary's Park, a wonderful green oasis. The city of Baltimore renovated the park with new plantings and new brickwork in 2011.

- Cut through the park wherever you feel inspired to do so and link up with N. Paca St. on the other side. When you reach N. Paca St., head right.

- You can't miss St. Mary's Spiritual Center and Mother Seton House on the right. The Mother Seton House was the home of the first native-born American canonized as a saint, Elizabeth Ann Seton. Adjacent to her home is St. Mary's Spiritual Center, birthplace of the oldest Catholic seminary in the country and Maryland's first college. Seton moved here in 1808 with her three daughters. On the day she arrived, the first bishop of the United States, John Carroll, dedicated the chapel behind her house. It was fortuitous timing. Here, Seton created and ran the country's first free school for girls. She also established the Sisters of Charity of St. Joseph, the country's first order of nuns. She stayed only a year, however, before moving to Emmitsburg, Maryland, to continue her work in association with what is today's Mount St. Mary's University, which graduated its first class in 1808. Canonization efforts for Seton began in 1907 and were completed in 1975.

  Also on the same grounds, the Seminary Chapel has been in continuous use for more than 200 years. It is the country's first example of neo-Gothic architecture and was designed by the celebrated French architect Maximilian Godefroy in 1808. It was here that Seton took her vows. The lower chapel was also the founding spot of the

Oblate Sisters of Providence, created in 1829 by Haitian immigrant Mary Elizabeth Lange, giving the Oblate Sisters the distinction of being the first African American Catholic community of nuns in the United States. The grounds, chapel, and Mother Seton House are all open for tours. Call for times and arrangements (see "Points of Interest" below).

- Across N. Paca St. from the Mother Seton House is George St. Take a quick detour up George St. to see some original 1800s row homes.

- Head back to N. Paca St. and go left. At 409 N. Paca St., you'll see the World Headquarters of Fluid Movement (fluidmovement.org). When Baltimorean and celebrated director John Waters commented, "It's as if every freak in the south was headed to New York, ran out of gas in Baltimore, and decided to stay," he may have had Fluid Movement in mind. The "freakiness" Fluid Movement produces is spectacular. Past performances have included water ballet, hula-hoop-athons, roller-skating ballets, and a celebration of the centennial of Baltimore's Great Fire featuring flamenco and funk "conflagrative interpretations."

- Continuing on to 323 N. Paca St., you'll come to a now defunct firehouse. Look for the interesting building behind the firehouse; the bottom three floors are boarded up, but pleasant domestic scenes have been painted around the windows of all three upper stories. The juxtaposition seems, somehow, to be a good metaphor for Baltimore itself.

- At 309 N. Paca St., you'll come to the St. Jude's Shrine, at the corner of W. Saratoga St. (the Shrine's physical address is 512 W. Saratoga St.). Established in 1917, the Shrine is under the direction of the Pallottine Fathers and Brothers, under the guidance of the Archbishop of Baltimore. Here people from all over the country offer petitions for prayer during the Perpetual Novena Services. A look inside reveals many prayers in the form of votive candles. If nothing else, there's something just downright cool in seeing the pilgrimage site for the patron saint of hopeless causes.

- You'll reach Lexington Market where N. Paca St. and W. Lexington St. meet. The fact that it's been continuously operated as a market for 220 years makes it the country's oldest. The area was once part of John Eager Howard's enormous estate. Upon his triumphant return from the battle places of the Revolutionary War, he okayed the donation of land for a farmers' market. For 20 years, farmers and merchants came from the surrounding areas and set up stalls, unloading their wagons after traveling for hours. In 1803, the first permanent structure was erected, a shed at Eutaw and Lexington. The place boomed thereafter. In 1822, U.S. Attorney General William Wirt wrote, "You may conceive the vast quantity of provisions that must be brought to this market when you are told that 60,000 people draw their daily supplies from it, which is more than twice as many people as there are in Washington, Georgetown, Alexandria and Richmond, all in one." In 1949, a massive fire broke out in the market and it was almost destroyed. But as it had been an integral part of local, regional, and national life for more than 150 years by then, its rebuilding was never really in doubt.

Lexington Market remains one of Baltimore's great local institutions. You can still get almost anything you need (chocolate, perfume, and socks, all in one place?), and the cacophony of sounds, smells, and sights makes dropping by an experience in and of itself. But as any self-respecting Baltimorean would, let's talk crab cakes. Many locals consider the cakes at Faidley's hands-down the best in the city, which makes them, by extension, the best in the world. The stall has been where you see it today since 1886 and is run by the fifth generation of the family. Whether they serve the best crab cakes in the city (or the world) isn't for me to say, but it's undoubtedly worth delving into the debate.

● You have several options here. After filling yourself at the market, either retrace your route back to your car in Seton Hill, take one of the many public-transport options at the market to your next destination, or take another walk; there are two along this route (see "Connecting the Walks" on the next page).

POINTS OF INTEREST (START TO FINISH)

St. Mary's Spritual Center & Historic Site/Mother Seton House stmarysspiritualcenter.org/mothersetonhouse.org, 600 N. Paca St., 410-728-6464 (central office)/410-523-3443 (Mother Seton House)

Fluid Movement fluidmovement.org, 409 N. Paca St.

St. Jude Shrine stjudeshrine.org, 512 W. Saratoga St., 410-685-6026

Lexington Market lexingtonmarket.com, 400 W. Lexington St., 410-685-6169

route summary

1. Start at Druid Hill Ave. and Orchard St.
2. Head southwest on Orchard St.
3. Turn left onto Pennsylvania Ave.
4. Turn left onto St. Mary St.
5. Cut through St. Mary's Park.
6. Turn right onto N. Paca St.
7. Turn left onto George St.
8. Return to N. Paca St. and go left.
9. Follow N. Paca St. to Lexington Market.

connecting the walks

When you turned left onto Pennsylvania Ave. from Orchard St., you could just as easily have gone right. Doing so would take you right into the Pennsylvania Avenue Heritage Trail (see Walk 17). The end point for this walk, Lexington Market, is also the starting point of Walk 13: Downtown: The Raven to the Ravens.

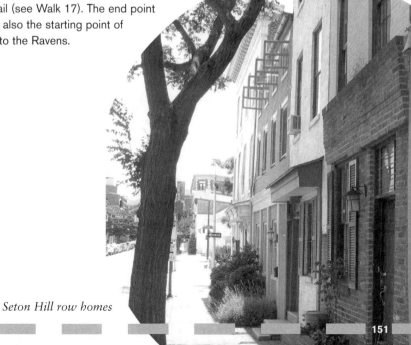

Seton Hill row homes

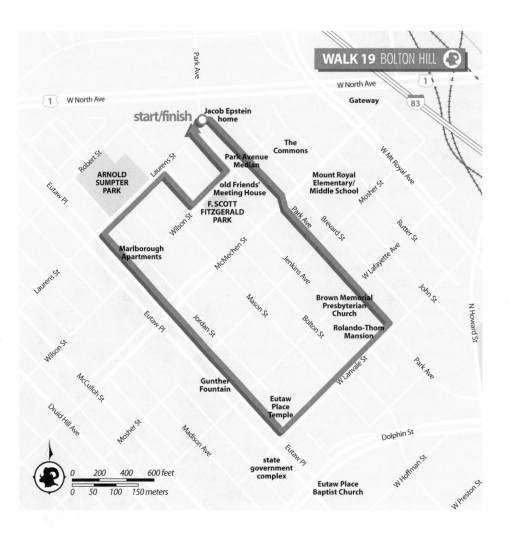

W North Ave

1

W North Ave

Gateway

83

Park Ave

start/finish

Jacob Epstein home

The Commons

W Mt Royal Ave

Robert St.

ARNOLD SUMPTER PARK

Laurens St.

Park Avenue Median

old Friends' Meeting House

Mount Royal Elementary/ Middle School

Mosher St.

Eutaw Pl

Wilson St.

F. SCOTT FITZGERALD PARK

Park Ave

Brevard St.

Rutter St.

W Lafayette Ave

Marlborough Apartments

McMechen St.

Jenkins Ave

John St

Laurens St.

Mason St.

Brown Memorial Presbyterian Church

N Howard St.

Eutaw Pl

Jordan St.

Bolton St.

Rolando-Thom Mansion

Wilson St.

W Lanvale St.

Park Ave

McCulloh St.

Gunther Fountain

Druid Hill Ave

Mosher St.

Madison Ave

Eutaw Place Temple

Eutaw Pl

Dolphin St

W Hoffman St.

W Preston St.

0   200   400   600 feet

0   50   100   150 meters

state government complex

Eutaw Place Baptist Church

19 BOLTON HILL: a Gallery of Luminaries

BOUNDARIES: **Park Ave., W. Lanvale St., Eutaw Pl., Laurens St., Bolton St., Wilson St.**
DISTANCE: **1.75 miles**
DIFFICULTY: **Easy**
PARKING: **Street parking all along route**
PUBLIC TRANSIT: **MTA bus #91 runs up and down Eutaw Pl.; MTA buses #5 and #13 stop on North Ave., near Park Ave.**

The Bolton Hill neighborhood has signified many things over the years—wealth, easy living, and a knack for attracting, rearing, and retaining an extraordinary collection of outsize personalities. Markers on today's Bolton Hill houses immortalize these personalities through the neighborhood's Blue Plaques program, modeled after a similar program in London. A century and a half ago, Bolton Hill's location a mile and a half from downtown made it a tough sell. But after the installation of a trolley line to serve the neighborhood, Bolton Hill was advertised as a special sort of paradise, removed from the hustle and bustle of the docks down by the harbor. Though it now sits in the middle of an expanded Baltimore City, Bolton Hill still retains a whiff of exclusivity. This walk takes in the faded (and not so faded) splendor of Bolton Hill's wonderful and unique brownstones and travels the paths of writers, artists, philosophers, and philanthropists, easily identified by the numerous historical markers. I encourage you to wander every side street in Bolton Hill for plentiful wonderful surprises. To see a complete list of who lived where, check out the Bolton Hill Association website at boltonhill.org.

● Heading west from I-83, exiting at North Ave., take the first left onto Park Ave. You will be in the 1700 block of Park Ave. The first plaque you can see is located at 1729 Park Ave., once the home of Jacob Epstein, a philanthropist who created the system of matching charitable grants. Note the extraordinary circular brick pattern in this house—a real beauty. Across the street, you can see carved Romanesque faces looming between the houses.

● Continue south on Park Ave. Straight ahead is the Park Avenue Median, a lovely stretch of green with fountains, benches, and flowers. It's a tough decision: whether to stick to the gorgeous brownstones or the greenery that splits them. 1500 Park is where six sons of John Prentiss Poe lived—all six were football stars at Princeton, a contrast to cousin Edgar Allan.

- The 1300 block of Park Avenue contains an embarrassment of historical riches: Among the more famous people to once call this block home: F. Scott Fitzgerald at #1307; Edith Hamilton, author of *The Greek Way,* at #1314; and Dr. Florence Rena Sabin, at #1325. Sabin's fame is more rightly honored in Colorado, however, as she was primarily responsible for the reform of that state's health laws and is today one of Colorado's two honorees in the U.S. Capitol's Statuary Hall.

- Approach W. Lafayette Ave. Continue on Park Ave., but if you want to see the home of Dr. Curt Richter, discoverer of the human biological clock, take a quick jaunt down W. Lafayette Ave. to #221. He lived in Baltimore until 1988, where he died at the age of 94.

  At the corner of W. Lafayette Ave. and Park Ave. is the beautiful limestone Brown Memorial Presbyterian Church, built in 1869. President McKinley once worshipped here, under the church's 11 Tiffany stained glass windows. Just beyond, at 1316 Park, is the administrative home of the Baltimore Choral Arts Society (performances take place elsewhere in the city).

- Turn right when you reach W. Lanvale St. At 127 W. Lanvale St. you'll find the home of Dr. Jesse Lazear, often called a "medical martyr" for his voluntary exposure to yellow fever–carrying mosquitoes. He proved the method of transmission but wound up dying in the process. 159 W. Lanvale St. is where Otto Mergenthaler lived and where he died in 1899. While his name might not ring a thousand bells, his invention of the Linotype revolutionized printing on a level almost comparable to Guttenberg's invention. Indeed, Thomas Edison described the Linotype as the "eighth wonder of the world."

- At 204 W. Lanvale St., between Jenkins Alley and Park Ave., you'll see the beautiful Gothic Rolando-Thom Mansion (built in 1848) that is now home to the Family and Children's Services of Central Maryland. 213 W. Lanvale St. was once the home of Col. Charles Marshall, Gen. Robert E. Lee's aide-de-camp at the surrender at Appomattox. 232 W. Lanvale St., at the corner of Bolton St., is where the discoverer of the anticoagulant heparin, Dr. William H. Howell, once resided. It is the neighborhood's oldest house, and one of the most beautiful.

- Continue on W. Lanvale St. You'll enter a great little park, notable for its three stone lions with their mouths agape and paws upraised. These lions were salvaged from the demolition of the old Calvert Street Bridge.

● You'll next reach Eutaw Pl., the largest road in Bolton Hill. To the left across Eutaw Pl. is the rather unattractive state government complex, built here because there wasn't room for this sprawling campus in Annapolis. Now, plans are afoot to move the state government buildings and employees to midtown. Something far more attractive than these boxy buildings is straight in front of you in the median on Eutaw Pl.: the Francis Scott Key Monument. Dedicated and built in 1907 by the French sculptor Marius Jean Antonin Mercié, the Key Monument is what F. Scott Fitzgerald referred to when recalling his fondness for Baltimore (see "Back Story" on page 156). It depicts Key in a small boat with attendant rower (the water that used to be here has, unfortunately, been drained) offering the star-spangled banner to a golden Columbia high atop four marble pillars. It's a beautiful and arresting piece of public art.

Two more striking buildings sit just to your right and to your left. On the right is the Byzantine Eutaw Place Temple. Architect Joseph Evans Sperry, who was also responsible for the Bromo Seltzer Tower, among other notable Baltimore buildings, designed the temple. It was built in 1892 for the Oheb Shalom congregation, who occupied it until moving in 1960, at which point the Prince Hall Masons purchased it. The great poet and Baltimorean Karl Shapiro was bar mitzvahed and married in this temple. Looking southeast to the next block, across Dolphin St., you can see the original Eutaw Place Baptist Church (1871). Its tower rises almost 200 feet. Architect of the Capitol Thomas Ustick Walter designed this church. Woodrow Wilson lived across the street, at 1210 Eutaw Pl., while he was earning his doctorate at Johns Hopkins. Those who knew him as a young man all remarked that he was nakedly ambitious and overly confident. But one wonders if even he

Eutaw Place Temple

Back Story

There are several locations in and around the city where F. Scott Fitzgerald fans can commune with the spirit of the great American writer. But it was from his residence at 1307 Park Ave. that he wrote the following: "Baltimore is warm but pleasant. I love it more than I thought—it is so rich with memories—it is nice to look up the street and see the statue of my great uncle Francis Scott Key and to know Poe is buried here and that many ancestors of mine have walked in the old town by the bay. I belong here, where everything is civilized and gay and rotted and polite. And I wouldn't mind a bit if in a few years Zelda & I could snuggle up together under a stone in some old graveyard here. That is really a happy thought and not melancholy at all." He also wrote much of the novel *Tender is the Night* here. Fitzgerald's wish to snuggle up with Zelda under a stone in a Baltimore graveyard didn't pan out. However, he's buried barely an hour away, in St. Mary's Catholic Church in Rockville, Maryland.

imagined that almost 30 years after studying at Hopkins, he would survive 46 ballots to win the Democratic nomination for president just a few blocks away at the Fifth Regiment Armory on Division St. Johns Hopkins University's first president and first director of the Johns Hopkins Hospital, the esteemed Daniel Coit Gilman, made his home at 1300 Eutaw Pl.

● Take a right on Eutaw Pl. Near the corner of W. Lafayette Ave. and Eutaw Pl. is the prominent and recently restored Gunther Fountain, originally displayed in 1876 as part of the Philadelphia Centennial Exposition. 1404 Eutaw Pl. was once the home of 19th-century poet Sidney Lanier, the first writer-in-residence at Johns Hopkins, now buried in Greenmount Cemetery (see Walk 21: Station North). You'll pass the beautiful Marlborough Apartments at 1701 Eutaw Pl.—here, sisters Claribel and Etta Cone displayed their vast collection of extraordinary 20th-century art, amassing more than 500 pieces by Henri Matisse, plus works by Cézanne, Gaguin, Picasso, and others. You can view a video re-creation of their apartments at the Baltimore Museum of Art (see Walk 25: Charles Village & JHU). The BMA also houses the bulk of the Cone sisters' collection, giving the museum the largest concentration of Matisse works in the world.

● Take a right onto Laurens St., passing nice row homes and eventually passing one of the last remaining signs of the old trolley line that used to service the neighborhood. This street was named for John Laurens, one of George Washington's officers.

● Take a right onto Bolton St. At the corner of Bolton St. and Wilson St., take a left and enjoy some shaded respite in the diminutive F. Scott Fitzgerald Park.

● Continuing east on Wilson St, pass Jenkins Alley and take a left onto Park Ave. You'll soon pass on the left some lovely condos inside the old Friends' Meeting House; the Friends Society of America (Quakers) have had an important presence in Baltimore for more than two centuries. If you drove, your car will be just up the block on Park Ave.

POINTS OF INTEREST (START TO FINISH)

Bolton Hill's Blue Plaques boltonhill.org/neighborhood/n_plaque.html
Brown Memorial Presbyterian Church 1316 Park Ave., 410-523-1542
Rolando-Thom Mansion 204 W. Lanvale St.
Francis Scott Key Monument Eutaw Pl. and W. Lanvale St.
Eutaw Place Temple 1307 Eutaw Pl.
Eutaw Place Baptist Church Dolphin St. and Eutaw St.

ROUTE SUMMARY

1. Begin in the 1700 block of Park Ave. and walk southeast.
2. Turn right onto W. Lanvale St.
3. Turn right onto Eutaw Pl.
4. Turn right onto Laurens St.
5. Turn right onto Bolton St.
6. Turn left onto Wilson St.
7. Turn left onto Park Ave.

CONNECTING THE WALKS

Two blocks south of the starting point to this walk is McMechen Street. Walk 20: Mount Royal begins on McMechen, just below W. Mount Royal Ave., three blocks northeast of Park Ave.

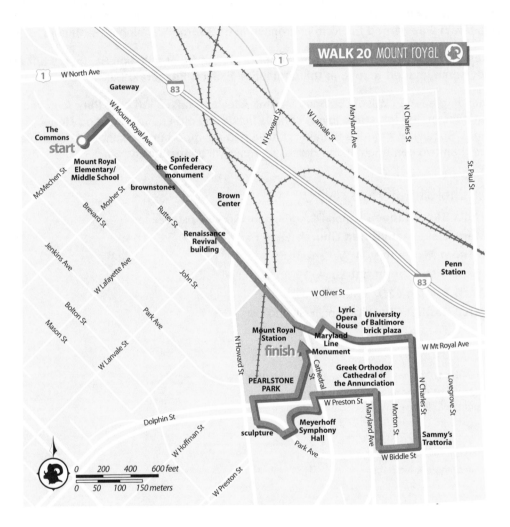

1 W North Ave

83 Gateway

1

W Mount Royal Ave

The Commons
start

Mount Royal Elementary/ Middle School

McMechen St

Mosher St

brownstones

Brevard St

Spirit of the Confederacy monument

Rutter St

Brown Center

Renaissance Revival building

Jenkins Ave

W Lafayette Ave

John St

Bolton St

Park Ave

Mason St

W Lanvale St

Dolphin St

W Hoffman St

W Preston St

N Howard St

N Howard St

W Lanvale St

Maryland Ave

N Charles St

St. Paul St

Penn Station

83

W Oliver St

Lyric Opera House

University of Baltimore brick plaza

Mount Royal Station
finish

Maryland Line Monument

Cathedral St

Greek Orthodox Cathedral of the Annunciation

PEARLSTONE PARK

W Preston St

sculpture

Meyerhoff Symphony Hall

Park Ave

W Biddle St

Maryland Ave

Morton St

N Charles St

Lovegrove St

W Mt Royal Ave

Sammy's Trattoria

0   200   400   600 feet

0   50   100   150 meters

20 MOUNT ROYAL: CULTURAL CAPITAL

BOUNDARIES: **Mount Royal Ave., Charles St., Biddle St., Cathedral St.**
DISTANCE: **1.6 miles**
DIFFICULTY: **Easy**
PARKING: **Street parking along route, much of it metered**
PUBLIC TRANSIT: **Mt. Royal/UB Light Rail; Cultural Center Light Rail; MTA buses #s 3, 11, 21, 61, and 64; Charm City Circulator Purple**

When it comes to being an arts and cultural center, Baltimore is in a tough spot. Washington, D.C., sits just 40 miles to the south, with its plethora of Smithsonian attractions. Likewise, New York City is only a few hours north. In 1991, then National Football League Commissioner Paul Tagliabue told a Baltimore reporter that the city "should build a museum" after Baltimore lost an expansion bid to replace the much-beloved Colts. The nasty and never forgotten implication was clear: the city didn't deserve football and probably needed some more cultural attractions, to boot. Well, nowadays, Baltimore does just fine in both categories, thank you very much. Despite being sandwiched between two cultural titans, Baltimore has gained a national reputation as a wonderful arts city, with a thriving music scene, a surfeit of galleries, and top-flight museums and theater. This walk takes in Baltimore's Cultural Capital. While by no means exhausting the city's cultural offerings, this walk through Mount Royal visits some of the most prominent. With the Maryland Institute College of Art, the University of Baltimore, an opera house, a symphony hall, a ton of restaurants, and a beautiful old train depot, Mount Royal lives up to its name. There's a ready supply of energy and bustle here. And for one extended weekend each July, the neighborhood hosts Artscape, the country's largest free arts festival. It's happening, man. Feel the energy.

● After getting off the JFX at North Ave., heading southwest, take the first left onto Park Ave. *Note:* just at the intersection of the off-ramp for the JFX and North Ave. is a beautiful 1903 bronze and granite monument to Colonel William Watson, who commanded the Baltimore Battalion and District of Columbia Volunteers during the Mexican-American War. Watson is remembered in the fourth verse of "Maryland, My Maryland," the state song: "Come! 'tis the red dawn of the day / Maryland! / Come with thy panoplied array / Maryland! / With Ringgold's spirit for the fray, / With Watson's blood at Monterey / With fearless Lowe and dashing May, / Maryland! My

Maryland!" When Park Ave. splits, keep left and take a left on McMechen St. Park anywhere near The Commons, the Maryland Institute College of Art's (MICA) dormitories, or Mount Royal Elementary/Middle School across the street. From your parking spot, walk east on McMechen St. until you soon reach the intersection with W. Mount Royal Ave. Across the street, you'll see the Gateway, MICA's apartment complex for students, designed specifically to accommodate artists and their need for studio space. Take a right onto W. Mount Royal Ave.

● This is a busy stretch of W. Mount Royal Ave., so it's not extremely pleasant initially. However, you'll soon see a nice green median to the left and some wonderful old turn-of-the-20th-century brownstones to the right, many of them sporting beautiful arched entranceways. To the left, you'll see a monument to the Confederacy, reflecting Maryland's tenuous nature during the Civil War: a border state, full of both loyalists and secessionists, part of the Union but allowing the continuation of slavery until 1864. This monument is known as the Spirit of the Confederacy. The pedestal reads "Gloria Victis," or "Glory to the Vanquished."

● Continuing on W. Mount Royal Ave., you'll soon come to two of MICA's main buildings; the contrast between them is striking. First, across W. Mount Royal Ave., after the intersection with W. Lafayette Ave., is the ultramodern Brown Center, looking like a steel parallelogram skeleton draped with translucent cloth. The building houses MICA's offices and studio space for its graphic design and interactive media programs. The architectural plans were drawn up using the same technology MICA students in the program will learn and employ. Almost directly across the street is MICA's 1907 Renaissance Revival building. It's as if the future stretches to meet the past. It's an appropriate analogy: MICA began in 1826, making it the country's oldest continuous degree-granting arts college. It has grown quite a bit over the years and is now nationally recognized as one of the best arts colleges in the United States. Its prestige is a reflection of its continued growth. But its long history helps to secure its place as a trendsetting college of the future.

● Continue on W. Mount Royal Ave., crossing W. Lanvale St. and continuing to the Light Rail tracks at the University of Baltimore stop. Looming ahead, down in a bowl to the right, is the magnificent Mount Royal Station. The B&O constructed this enormous Romanesque edifice in 1896 as part of its efforts to improve and upgrade its

Baltimore Belt Line passenger service to New York. It was at Mount Royal that the B&O installed the country's first railway-electrification system, allowing trains to move by electricity as opposed to coal or diesel. MICA purchased the station, as well as surrounding acreage, in 1964, a dozen years before Mount Royal Station's designation as a National Historic Landmark. Today, the building houses MICA's school of sculpture, an art gallery, and studio and classroom space. You can descend the stairs to see the old train shed. But access to inside space might be restricted, depending on school hours and usage.

● Return to street level. Take note of the prominent statue on Cathedral St. at W. Mount Royal Ave.: This is the Maryland Line Monument. It's a 60-foot column topped by the Goddess of Liberty, dedicated in 1901. Liberty holds the Declaration of Independence in one hand and a laurel wreath in the other. Maryland's Revolutionary-era militias were reputed to be among the colonies' fiercest, gaining them the moniker, courtesy of George Washington, "The Old Line," meaning a force that could not be breached. (It is this that gives Maryland its nickname "The Old Line State" and not, as is generally presumed, the Mason-Dixon Line.) This monument honors the Old Line, known as the The Bayonets of the Continental Army.

● Cross Cathedral St. and head to the Lyric Opera House. Built in 1894, just two years before Mount Royal Station, the opera house began its life as The Music Hall with a performance by the Boston Symphony Orchestra. It has been updated and enhanced many times over the past 120 years, but a 2011 renovation allowed the Lyric to call itself a truly modern venue while still retaining much of its historical flavor. A new crosswalk built behind the stage allows actors to move to either side of the stage undetected by the

Mount Royal brownstones

Back Story

Artscape began in 1982, when people questioned whether city-dwellers in general and Baltimoreans in particular were interested in gathering during the swelter of July to watch street performers and visual artists hawking their wares. There was real concern in the beginning as to whether famously segregated Baltimoreans would come together to share a common experience. The good news was that it worked then—and it works now. Artscape today is a celebration of Baltimore's quirkiness and unique character, annually attracting more than 350,000 attendees over three days from as wide a socioeconomic and ethnic swath as seems possible. Sculpture, arts and crafts, music, food, opera, theater, film, dance: it's all here and all on display. Seeing Ray Charles or Aretha Franklin perform for free in front of Mount Royal Station? Little could be better, despite the summer heat.

audience; before the renovation, such a move meant a cramped and uncomfortable trip beneath the stage, a logistical nightmare. The stage itself has grown much larger with the renovation as well, increasing in both height and depth. The orchestra pit has also been improved. There are few theatergoers or music lovers in Baltimore who have not seen at least one show at the Lyric; with the new improvements, the experience promises to be even more memorable.

● With the Lyric Opera House on your left, cross Maryland Ave. You're now in the heart of the downtown campus of the University of Baltimore, best known for its law school. You'll see UB's new student center across W. Mount Royal Ave., to the right. The plans for this building caused much consternation in 2003–04, when it was learned that they included the demolition of the 1915 Tudor-style Odorite building (beautiful building, not-so-beautiful name). The name Odorite, of course, reflected the previous tenants: a janitorial-supply company. However, the building itself was originally the home of the Monumental Motor Car Company and was one of the last remaining car showroom buildings that used to be ubiquitous along Mount Royal Ave. It was here that midcentury Baltimoreans went to buy their Packards and Chevys and Studebakers. Despite the understandable lament from local preservationists, many concede that the student center is a lovely replacement. It's most notable for its glass, diamond-shaped stairway enclosure and its curved rooftop structures, which house a theater.

To your left, in the University of Baltimore brick plaza, is sculptor Moses J. Ezekiel's 1921 Edgar Allan Poe monument. The Poe monument spent its first 60 years in Wyman Park, but it was brought here in 1983.

● Follow the street to the end of the block and go right on N. Charles St. Charles Street is for many (including me) a favorite street in Baltimore. It's Charm City's Champs-Élysées or Las Ramblas. Stretching all the way from I-95 in South Baltimore to beyond the city limits up to Towson in the north, Charles St. is stocked with eateries, shops, historic sites, plazas, businesses, museums, and all the people-watching one could ever wish for. The section of N. Charles St. in this walk's description is notable for its many brownstones and myriad eating options. One of my favorites is Sammy's Trattoria, located at the corner of N. Charles St. and W. Biddle St.

● No doubt you've noticed several interesting and enticing sites in the last block, but don't worry—in every case, these are covered in nearby walks. For example, Penn Station is in Walk 21: Station North, and the Beaux Arts Belvedere, looming ahead to the left—it's unmistakable with its unique mansard roof—is in Walk 16: Mount Vernon. Save these wonderful, close-by sights. For now, take a right on W. Biddle St. and follow it to the next block, Maryland Ave. At Maryland Ave., take a right.

Note: for a quick and easy diversion, first go left on W. Biddle St. and follow it five blocks (it will have become E. Biddle St.) to two addresses: 212 E. Biddle, once the home of author Gertrude Stein, and 215 E. Biddle, the home of Wallis Warfield, whose allure was enough to make King Edward VIII abdicate his throne to marry her, thereby making her the Duchess of Windsor.

● Cross the street at the next block, W. Preston St., and take a few steps to the left. There you'll see the wonderful Greek Orthodox Cathedral of the Annunciation, built in 1889. It's a grand old stone Byzantine building, which would be out of place if not for its circular appearance, shared by both the University of Baltimore Student Center roof and the nearby Meyerhoff Symphony Hall. Across the street, at 45 W. Preston, is the Baltimore Theatre Project, a 40-year-old institution that began with free shows and now offers terrific theater and dance. The attractive building that houses the Baltimore Theatre Project dates to 1887.

● Continue on W. Preston to Cathedral St. and cross to see the Meyerhoff Symphony Hall, home of another beloved cultural institution, the Baltimore Symphony Orchestra (BSO). The Meyerhoff was built in 1982, on the heels of Baltimore's burgeoning renaissance emanating from the restyled Inner Harbor. If Baltimore was to be a world-class city, it needed a world-class symphony hall. And that is precisely what the Meyerhoff is. The most striking aspect of the Meyerhoff is that it was built without any flat walls or 90-degree angles. Curves dominate the building, inside and out, providing for an amazing acoustic experience. Today, the Meyerhoff hosts not only the BSO, but also an eclectic collection of acts from all over the musical map, as well as stars from the world of comedy and visual arts.

● Walk around the Meyerhoff, keeping it on your left and W. Preston St. on your right, until you reach Park Ave. In front of you are a small green space with a modernist sculpture, N. Howard St., and the fascinating fortress-looking Fifth Regiment Armory looming ahead. On the first floor of the building, there's a drill hall that measures 200 by 300 feet; here, Woodrow Wilson, who once lived a few blocks away in Bolton Hill, was selected to be the Democratic nominee for the presidential election of 1912.

● Cross W. Preston St. and enter Pearlstone Park; you'll see Mount Royal Station ahead.

● From Mount Royal Station, you can retrace your steps along W. Mount Royal Ave. back to where you began, at McMechen St. However, it's easy to link with several other nearby walks. In fact, you are within a few blocks of two of them. See "Connecting the Walks" on the next page.

POINTS OF INTEREST (START TO FINISH)

Maryland Institute College of Art mica.edu, 1300 W. Mount Royal Ave., 410-669-9200

Mount Royal Station www.mica.edu/browse_art/mount_royal_station.html, 1300 W. Mount Royal Ave., 410-669-9200

Lyric Opera House lyricoperahouse.com, 110 W. Mount Royal Ave., 410-685-5086

University of Baltimore ubalt.edu, 1420 N. Charles St., 410-837-4200

Sammy's Trattoria sammystrattoria.com, 1200 N. Charles St., 410-837-9999

Greek Orthodox Cathedral of the Annunciation goannun.org, 24 W. Preston St., 410-727-2641

Baltimore Symphony Orchestra/Meyerhoff Symphony Hall bsomusic.org, 1212 Cathedral St., 410-783-8000

Fifth Regiment Armory 219 29th Division St., 410-576-6097

route summary

1. Begin on McMechen St. and walk northeast to W. Mount Royal Ave.
2. Take a right on W. Mount Royal Ave.
3. Continue on W. Mount Royal Ave. past the Light Rail tracks.
4. Descend the hill to Mount Royal Station.
5. Return to W. Mt. Royal Ave. and cross Cathedral St.
6. Continue on W. Mount Royal Ave., across Maryland Ave.
7. Take a right onto N. Charles St.
8. Take a right onto W. Biddle St.
9. Take a right onto Maryland Ave.
10. Take a left onto W. Preston St.
11. Cross Cathedral St. and Preston St. and enter Pearlstone Park.
12. Walk through the park to W. Mount Royal Ave.
13. Retrace your steps to McMechen St.

connecting the walks

To take Walk 19: Bolton Hill, simply continue on McMechen St. past where you parked to Park Ave. You can reach Walk 16: Mount Vernon by going south on Charles St.

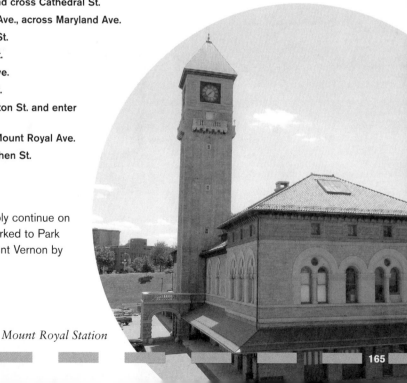

Mount Royal Station

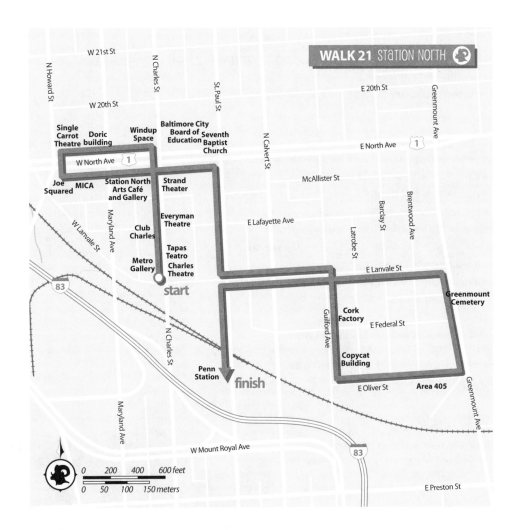

W 21st St

N Howard St

W 20th St

N Charles St

St. Paul St

E 20th St

Greenmount Ave

E North Ave

N Calvert St

Single
Carrot
Theatre

Doric
building

Windup
Space

Baltimore City
Board of
Education

Seventh
Baptist
Church

W North Ave

McAllister St

Joe
Squared

MICA

Station North
Arts Café
and Gallery

Strand
Theater

Barclay St

Brentwood Ave

E Lafayette Ave

Club
Charles

Everyman
Theatre

Latrobe St

E Lanvale St

W Lanvale St

Maryland Ave

Metro
Gallery

Tapas
Teatro
Charles
Theatre

start

Greenmount
Cemetery

Guilford Ave

Cork
Factory

E Federal St

N Charles St

Penn
Station

finish

Copycat
Building

E Oliver St

Area 405

Greenmount Ave

Maryland Ave

W Mount Royal Ave

E Preston St

0   200   400   600 feet

0   50   100   150 meters

21 STATION NORTH: AN OFFICIAL ARTS & ENTERTAINMENT DISTRICT

BOUNDARIES: **W. North Ave., Greenmount Ave., N. Charles St., Penn Station and tracks**
DISTANCE: **3.2 miles**
DIFFICULTY: **Moderate to strenuous**
PARKING: **Street parking all along route**
PUBLIC TRANSIT: **Amtrak and Light Rail at Penn Station; Charm City Circulator Purple and MTA buses #s 3, 11, and 64 all stop near Penn Station; MTA bus #36 runs north–south along Guilford Ave.; MTA bus #13 runs east–west along North Ave.; MTA bus #8 runs north–south along Greenmount Ave.**

There's a dividing line near Penn Station. To the immediate south lie Mount Royal and Mount Vernon, two of the more visited and sought-after neighborhoods in central Baltimore. To the immediate north and west are the neighborhoods of Charles North, Greenmount West, and Barclay, now known collectively as Station North. Not only has the train station served as a physical boundary, but it has also functioned as something of a psychological one. The streets wrapping around Penn Station to the north and west suffer from higher crime rates and more pronounced poverty than those south. There are still problems, to be sure, but an amazing transformation has taken place in Station North in the past decade. However, it has not been the type of gentrification we've seen in so many other places in which urban pioneers snap up abandoned old, but beautiful, properties and, in the process of improving derelict blocks, also price out locals who have made their homes in the area for generations. The newcomers in Station North, by contrast, have been largely young artists, drawn by the area's official designation as an Arts and Entertainment District, the city's first. The primary result of that 2002 designation has meant that several abandoned warehouses have been rezoned for residential use; artists looking for cheap accommodations and performance space have found paradise in these old buildings. The resulting changes have been as swift as they have been dramatic: a surfeit of performance space and art gallery showings, and the inevitable small businesses to serve the influx of people and energy. Indeed, it's an exciting time for Station North, and its recent transformation is great for Baltimore, further enhancing its deserved reputation as a town with a terrific arts scene. In this walk, take in the artistic highlights of

Station North, plus the station that gives it its name and the city's Père-Lachaise: Greenmount Cemetery, home to many of Baltimore's deceased elite.

Note: Some sections of this walk traverse blighted areas where some walkers might feel uncomfortable, primarily the eastern edges near Greenmount Ave., E. Lanvale St., and E. Oliver St. Use common sense. This route is also drivable.

● Begin where Falls Rd. ends at Maryland Ave. Cross Maryland Ave., and Falls Rd. becomes Lanvale St. You will see Pennsylvania Station (just Penn Station to locals) to your right. You'll end up there, so for now take the first left onto N. Charles St. Immediately, you are on one of the major strips that earns the neighborhood its Arts and Entertainment designation. On the left, on the corner of Lanvale St. and N. Charles St., is the Metro Gallery, which functions as art gallery and performance space (and has an extensive selection of beer and wine). The gallery also hosts the Videopolis film festival, which shows, for free, nontraditional shorts and feature-length films during the annual four-day Maryland Film Festival. On the other side of the street is the esteemed Charles Theatre, one of the venues that hosts the film festival, which attracts not only local film and TV personalities, such as Barry Levinson, Matthew Porterfield, David Simon, and John Waters, but also national stars. Festival events are held throughout Station North (for more information, visit mdfilmfest. com). The Charles Theatre building is an 1892 Beaux Arts beauty that was originally a cable car barn. In 1939, it became the Times Theatre, Baltimore's first all-newsreel movie house. It became the Charles in 1959 and spent the next 40 years as a single-screen theater. Now there are five screens, and Baltimoreans know it as the place to go not only for first-run Hollywood flicks, but also for foreign, classic, and revival films. Connected to the Charles is the great tapas restaurant Tapas Teatro. If you prefer crepes, check out Sofi's, on the north side of the Charles. Across the street is the cozy Club Charles, a bar John Waters has been known to frequent.

On the corner of the block, just before E. Lafayette Ave., is the longtime home of the Everyman Theatre. The resident actors who make up the Everyman are known as some of the best in the city, and they have been offering classic and original shows at affordable prices for more than 20 years. During a time when so many smaller repertories are closing up shop, the Everyman Theatre's expansion is a testament to its quality and the beloved status it holds for many Baltimoreans. By the time you read this, however, the production company will have probably already moved to its new $17 million space on the Westside (see Walk 13: Downtown: The Raven to the Ravens).

● Stay on N. Charles and cross E. Lafayette Ave. (If you're interested, you can take a quick detour by taking a right onto E. Lafayette to the Schuler School of Fine Arts and Gallery, just to the right at #7 and #9 E. Lafayette. The atelier school has been there for 50 years and focuses on the techniques and styles of the old masters.) If you come to this section of N. Charles St. at night, you can witness the full effect of "glassphalt," which is created when conventional asphalt is mixed with small amounts of glass. The result is beautiful—car headlights make the road glitter like diamonds. At 1800 N. Charles is the 1930 Walbert building. You'll see many small businesses on both sides of the street, including the popular Bohemian Coffee House and the Station North Arts Café and Gallery. Next door is the Strand Theater, "dedicated to providing opportunities for women artists, writers, designers and directors." Unfortunately, the Hexagon gallery and performance space, two doors north, closed in July 2011.

● Reach and then cross W. North Ave. At 10–12 W. North Ave. (on the corner of N. Charles St. and W. North Ave.) is the Windup Space. This performance space/gallery/bar has garnered a lot of attention and offers a plethora of events. Check out the website for more: thewindupspace.com. The Cyclops art gallery and bookstore is to the left, at the corner of W. North Ave. and Maryland Ave.

● Continue on W. North Ave. by crossing Maryland Ave. (and check out that gorgeous little Doric beauty on the corner—a little slice of Athens in Station North). Three doors down is Westnorth Studio, the home and

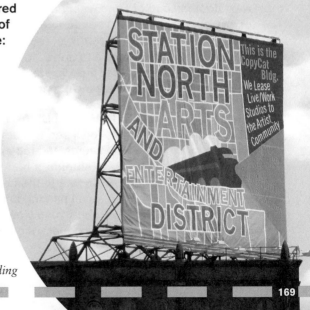

Station North billboard atop the Copycat building

studio of artist roycrosse. Continue to the end of the block to visit the Single Carrot Theatre and the Load of Fun Gallery.

"The day is coming when a single carrot, freshly observed, will set off a revolution," said painter Paul Cézanne. The Single Carrot Theatre, as much as any ensemble or arts organization, is responsible for Station North's revolution. Year after year it garners Best of Baltimore raves and has attracted national media attention. The story of how it wound up in Charm City is pretty cool too: a group of University of Colorado grads set out to create a theatre company and searched for the best place to do it. Starting with a list of 50 American locations, they narrowed the list to four based on a number of variables and ended up in Baltimore. J. Buck Jabaily, principal in the theater, said, "The thing that really impressed us was the openness of the Baltimore theater community. We didn't get that feeling anywhere else." Also important, of course, were cost of living and public support for the arts: because Station North rents are cheap and because of the city's and state's commitments to tax incentives thanks to the Arts and Entertainment designation, the Single Carrot wound up in the ex-garage on North Ave. Since its arrival, it has won over legions of fans with its emphasis on socially challenging work and its enthusiastic support of young artists.

Next door is Load of Fun Gallery and Load of Fun Theatre (LOF/t), home to a plethora of arts opportunities and happenings. There's the gallery, for one, showcasing both established and emerging artists. The space also hosts the wonderful and unique In-Flight Theater, trapeze and aerial apparatus shows like few you've seen before, as well as the Heralds of Hope Theater troupe and the Glass Mind Theater troupe. In other words, there is always something happening at the LOF/t.

● The end of the block is N. Howard St. Turn around and cross W. North Ave., keeping N. Howard St. on your right. You'll see two adjoining businesses: the über-popular Joe Squared, with its musical events and full menu, complete with its award-winning pizza; next door is the Hour Haus studios, a performance and recording space for musicians in a building that was once home to the headquarters of the Ma & Pa (Maryland and Pennsylvania) Railroad. A small parking area separates Joe Squared from the next up: an old Jos. A Bank warehouse now owned and operated by the Maryland Institute College of Art (MICA). As the country's oldest continuously operating degree-granting arts institution, MICA's presence in Station North is not only apropos, but is yet one more stabilizing presence along North Ave.

- Continue on W. North Ave., heading east. When you pass Maryland Ave. and then the McDonald's, look for the forlorn Parkway Theatre building on the right at 5 W. North Ave. The old theater dates to 1915 and was built as a vaudeville theater, holding more than one thousand seats. But as vaudeville faded, changes were made to the theater to make it a movie house, which it was for decades. It's something of a miracle that the place still stands; all too often, wonderful old buildings deemed to have outlived their usefulness are torn down. Plans are now afoot to revitalize and reuse the building.

- Stay on W. North Ave. to St. Paul St. Across W. North Ave., you'll see the beautiful Gothic limestone 1845 Seventh Baptist Church. Looming over the slight rise above North Ave. to the right of the church is the impressive columnar Baltimore City Board of Education building. Follow St. Paul St. south. Like much of St. Paul St. elsewhere in the city, it is flanked here by some impressive 19th- and early 20th-century town homes.

- Take a left onto E. Lanvale St. Follow it to Guilford Ave. and take a right. The last building on the left side of this block is the Cork Factory building, another central piece of Station North's transformation. And just beyond it, across Federal St. at 1501 Guilford Ave., is the 1890s Copycat building, so named for the large Copycat printing company billboard that stood on its roof—today, it has been replaced with the quickly becoming iconic Station North billboard. The original owner of both buildings was the Crown Cork & Seal Company. Today, the buildings are artists' residences and are full of open and airy performance spaces. The Copycat Theatre, for instance, operates out of the Copycat warehouse, as did the popular Wham City Collective, an artists group. Before the Arts and Entertainment designation came to Station North, clearing the way for tax incentives and rezoning, the residential artist squatters in these buildings were living there illegally. Now, all is on the up and up. Recent rumors of sales and rehabs have some residents afraid they will be priced out. Stay tuned. A possibility for displaced or incoming artists is the old Lebow Clothing Factory building, just behind the Cork & Seal buildings.

Back Story

Among the luminaries buried at Greenmount Cemetery is the first writer-in-residence of Johns Hopkins University, Sidney Lanier. To show his appreciation for the appointment, Lanier penned the "Ode to the Johns Hopkins University," in which he writes: "To walk familiar citizen of the town, / Bring Tolerance, that can kiss and disagree, / Bring Virtue, Honor, Truth, and Loyalty, / Bring Faith that sees with undissembling eyes, / Bring all large Loves and heavenly Charities, / Till man seem less a riddle unto man / And fair Utopia less Utopian, / And many peoples call from shore to shore, / 'The world has bloomed again, at Baltimore!'"

● Continue on Guilford Ave. to a left onto E. Oliver St., just before the Guilford Ave. bridge. Be aware: this block of E. Oliver contains some urban blight: abandoned and boarded-up houses and trash-choked lots. Use common sense here. That said, you're very close to one of Station North's successful and ambitious reclamation projects, Area 405, at 405 E. Oliver St. This 66,000-square-foot warehouse is 150 years old and served in its lifetime as a brewery, an industrial-equipment maker, and a window blind manufacturer. It is now one of the main artist-owned spaces in the district. Area 405's mission includes functioning as a promotion venue for artists throughout the Mid-Atlantic. You'll find new construction at 440 E. Oliver: the $15 million City Arts Apartments and Gallery, more living and performance space for resident artists.

● E. Oliver St. ends at Greenmount Ave. at an impressive place: the Greenmount Cemetery. The first thing about Greenmount Cemetery is its striking entrance: dark stone and wrought iron gates, giving it an appropriately Gothic feel. Like many old cemeteries, Greenmount is a beauty, full of exquisite memorials, statuary, and a stunning 150-year-old chapel. Inside, you'll find a collection of people as eclectic as the city itself. Established in 1838 and placed on the National Register of Historic Places in 1980, its first interment was for 2-year-old Olivia Cushing Whitridge. Over the years, 65,000 others joined her, including eight Maryland governors and eight Baltimore mayors. Major Baltimore benefactors such as Johns Hopkins, Henry

Walters, and Enoch Pratt are here, as are a slew of generals; Napoléon Bonaparte's sister-in-law; the co-conspirators in Abraham Lincoln's assassination, including Johns Wilkes Booth; and circus performer Johnny Eck, aka King of the Freaks, born without a lower half. If this were a dinner party, you'd never want to leave. Walking tours can be arranged. For contact information, see "Points of Interest" below and check out the cemetery's excellent website for history, maps, and other useful information.

● After Greenmount Cemetery, you'll want to head to this walk's final destination: Penn Station. The quickest way to get there is to take Greenmount Ave. three blocks north from the cemetery entrance at Oliver St. to E. Lanvale St. and head left (west) about eight blocks to St. Paul St. and go left. Just after the St. Paul St. bridge, you can take a right into Penn Station.

● Two rail structures preceded Penn Station at its location: the Northern Central Railway (1873) and the Charles Street Union Station (1886), which was demolished in 1910 to clear the way for the station that still serves central Baltimore today. The Union Station was built in 1911 for the Pennsylvania Railroad in a gorgeous Beaux Arts style out of granite and terra-cotta and was renamed Pennsylvania Station in 1928. When it was first completed, civic pride swelled. Gamble Latrobe, the superintendent of the Pennsylvania Railroad, boasted: "There is not a better railroad station in Philadelphia, in New York or in the country than this, and it all belongs to Baltimore." Today, Penn Station generally ranks in the top 10 passenger stations in America in terms of passengers served, with roughly 2 million annually and more than 150 trains daily.

Before you head inside the lovely station, you will undoubtedly see the still controversial *Male/Female* sculpture out front. Whether you find this an interesting and good piece of public art or an abomination is up to you. Either way, you'll have plenty of supporters for your view. Sculptor Jonathan Borofsky created this 51-foot statue out of aluminum in 2004. There's little question that its modern sensibility clashes rather mightily with the historic structure it fronts (somewhat like I. M. Pei's glass pyramids in front of the Louvre, one supposes); whether that creates an interesting and admirable duality—such is the piece's central theme—or simply an eyesore has been debated since the day it was erected. Whatever your decision, make sure to head inside; the station has been refurbished in recent years and its internal appearance today is much as it was 100 years ago. It really is a lovely building; look up at the ceiling when you enter to see the massive skylights.

POINTS OF INTEREST (START TO FINISH)

Maryland Film Festival mdfilm-fest.com, 410-752-8083

Greenmount Cemetery greenmountcemetery.com, 1501 Greenmount Ave., 410-539-0641

Penn Station 1500 N. Charles St.

Note: Most of the points of interest in this walk are gallery/performance space mixed with artists' residences, as well as small businesses that host public art happenings, all noted within the text. For a comprehensive listing that is kept up-to-date, visit stationnorth.org. There you will find lots of information on the locations noted here.

ROUTE SUMMARY

1. Start on N. Charles St. at E. Lanvale St. and head north.
2. Cross W. North Ave. eastbound and turn left onto W. North Ave. westbound.
3. Cross W. North Ave. westbound at N. Howard St. and turn left onto W. North Ave. eastbound.
4. Turn right onto St. Paul St.
5. Turn left onto E. Lanvale St.
6. Turn right onto Guilford Ave.
7. Turn left onto E. Oliver St.
8. Enter Greenmount Cemetery from Greenmount Ave.
9. Go north on Greenmount Ave.
10. Turn left onto E. Lanvale St.
11. Turn left onto St. Paul St.
12. Turn right into Penn Station.

CONNECTING THE WALKS

Walk 22: Falls Road Turnpike ends where this walk begins, at Falls Rd. just south of Maryland Ave. Walk 20: Mount Royal is just south of Penn Station, and Walk 16: Mount Vernon is just a few blocks south of Penn Station.

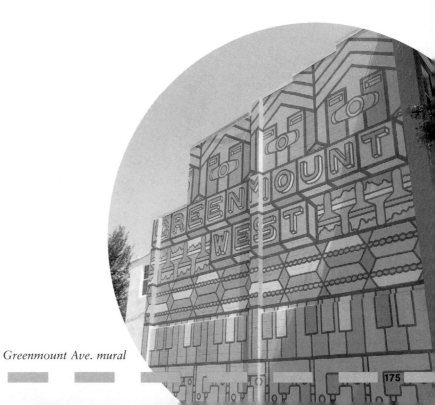

Greenmount Ave. mural

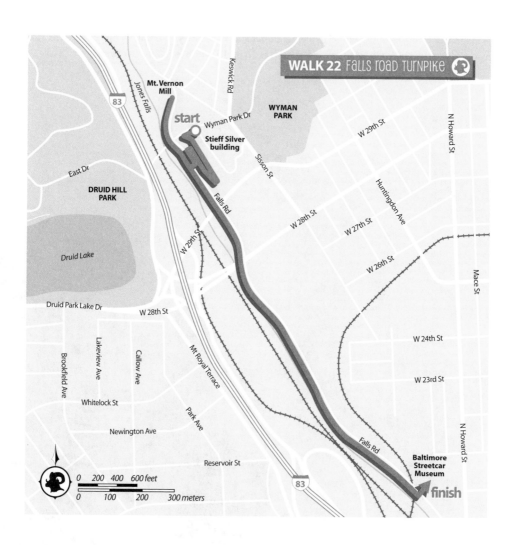

Mt. Vernon
Mill

Keswick Rd

**WYMAN
PARK**

W 29th St

N Howard St

start

Wyman Park Dr

**Stieff Silver
building**

Sisson St

Huntingdon Ave

**DRUID HILL
PARK**

East Dr

Falls Rd

W 28th St

W 27th St

W 26th St

Mace St

W 29th St

Druid Lake

Druid Park Lake Dr

W 28th St

W 24th St

Lakeview Ave

Callow Ave

Mt Royal Terrace

W 23rd St

Brookfield Ave

Whitelock St

Park Ave

Newington Ave

N Howard St

Falls Rd

**Baltimore
Streetcar
Museum**

Reservoir St

0   200   400   600 feet
0   100   200   300 meters

finish

22 Falls road Turnpike: YOU'D Hardly Know IT'S Here

BOUNDARIES: **Falls Rd., Jones Falls Trail**
DISTANCE: **1.8 miles**
DIFFICULTY: **Easy**
PARKING: **At Boy Scout Park**
PUBLIC TRANSIT: **MTA bus #98 (Hampden Shuttle) stops near Boy Scout Park at Keswick Rd. and Pacific Ave.**

Most Baltimore-area commuters know Falls Rd.; it stretches from midtown all the way through northern Baltimore County virtually to Pennsylvania. While these upper reaches are often spectacularly beautiful as the two-lane road winds its way through bucolic countryside, Falls Road in the city, while still lovely in places, sometimes fails to present its best face. The road—still just two lanes—is urbanized as it snakes through Hampden, but then it does something unexpected (and it's here that many Baltimoreans become unaware of its continued existence): it plunges into deep woods speckled with old mills and runs alongside its namesake, the Jones Falls. It was along the Jones Falls that abolitionist Elisha Tyson started a milling business in the 1790s. Tyson was a true philanthropist, with a special interest in the disenfranchised: the poor, the working class, African Americans. He then turned his attention to the creation of the Falls Road Turnpike along an old American Indian trail. This turnpike connected his Woodberry mill to others along the Jones Falls. As noted, many Baltimore drivers know Falls Road. But Tyson's portion—the original portion—is still shrouded in a somewhat mysterious aura: even though you're in the middle of the city, a stroll through here transports you a century or two back in time (assuming, of course, you can ignore the massive Jones Falls Expressway ramp above you nearby).

● Begin this walk on the portion of the Jones Falls Trail (JFT) where it intersects with Boy Scout Park. (Before you head down the JFT, take a quick glance across the park to the iconic Stieff Silver building; this 1920s beauty is on the National Register of Historic Places and was once home to the silver manufacturing giant. Now, it houses the Advanced Technology Laboratory of the Johns Hopkins University.) At the edge of the park, to the left of Wyman Park Dr., you'll see signs for the JFT pointing you toward Johns Hopkins University, Wyman Park, and the Inner Harbor. Follow the JFT as it switchbacks down the hill and dumps you out onto Falls Rd.

● Cross Falls Rd. to view Round Falls, a scenic view indicative of the Jones Falls' potential (and current) splendor. While many point to the Patapsco River, the Jones Falls is, in reality, Baltimore's main waterway, cleaving the city more or less right down the middle from just south of Lake Roland on the city/county line all the way to the Inner Harbor. The river is in some ways a microcosm of the city itself: exceedingly beautiful in spots, terribly neglected in others. An overturned and discarded shopping cart in the middle of the river may very well serve as a perch for a magnificent grey heron; an eroded bank speckled with storm-water-runoff detritus might also serve as a breeding ground for bullfrogs, snakes, turtles, or beavers. Because of the river's geographic location and where it spills its waters, its condition determines, to a large extent, the health of the city's natural spaces overall.

● With Round Falls to your back and Falls Rd. in front of you, head left. *Note:* there is no sidewalk here, so take caution. There is plenty of room on the road, however, and the distance to your destination is just a few hundred yards away. On your way, look for the remains of a water-driven mill wheel that operated until the 1920s, just above the Jones Falls underneath the first bridge you pass under (Wyman Park Dr.).

● Looming to the left, you'll see the Mt. Vernon Mill. You'll see signs marking the mill "1873" and "1879." It is here, at Mt. Vernon Mill No. 1 and No. 2, that Elisha Tyson's original gristmill stood. Mill No. 1 began life in 1847 as a cotton mill, contributing to the Jones Falls Valley's status as the world's largest producer of cotton duck (see Walk 28: Woodberry). The buildings you see about you now are listed on the National Register of Historic Places and date from 1845 to 1918. Most prominent are the three-story brick Mill Building (1873), the two-story L-shaped Picker House (1873), the two-story brick Store House (1881–82), and a concrete warehouse (1918). Ambitious rehabilitation plans are afoot—much work had already been accomplished by 2012— and include a $40 million renovation that will result in office space, apartments, and restaurants. Many of the mill windows were bricked over, and plans include restoring them to their original 19th-century appearance. The overall rehabilitation project incorporates green building and includes a plan to restore the Jones Falls in the immediate area and provide public water access. When you've taken a good look at the mill complex, return the way you came down Falls Rd. When you reach the overlook for Round Falls again, a sidewalk (part of the JFT) allows for an easier amble.

- Continue along the JFT, with the Jones Falls to your right, until you reach the Baltimore Streetcar Museum at 1901 Falls Rd. This remains one of Baltimore's lesser-known museums because of its obscure location, but its popularity has been growing in recent years—for good reason. In the Trolley Theatre, originally housed in the Baltimore City Life Museums, you can view a film about streetcars and their prominence in the life of Baltimore. And, of course, you can peruse the museum's trolley collection. Some highlights include a 1944 Pullman; a 1902 12-bench open car, perfect for steamy summer rides; an 1896 nine-bench open car; an 1880 passenger car from the United Railways and Electric Company; a gaslight fixture; and many more streetcars and trolley memorabilia. Many of the cars you see used to run the network of streetcar lines that allowed Baltimore to expand from a few square miles concentrated around the harbor to include once far-flung suburbs (now city neighborhoods) such as Bolton Hill and Roland Park.

- You can either turn around and retrace your steps back to Boy Scout Park or, my recommendation, stitch this walk together with Station North (see "Connecting the Walks" on the next page). To do that, continue on the JFT as it passes under the North Ave. and Howard St. bridges, and then rises to meet Maryland Ave.

POINTS OF INTEREST (START TO FINISH)

Mt. Vernon Mill Complex millno1.com, 3000 Falls Rd., 410-327-3200

Baltimore Streetcar Museum baltimorestreetcar.org, 1901 Falls Rd., 410-547-0264

route summary

1. Start at Boy Scout Park.
2. Follow the Jones Falls Trail (JFT) down the hill to Falls Rd.
3. Visit Round Falls.
4. Go north on Falls Rd. to the Mt. Vernon Mill complex.
5. Go south on Falls Rd. to the Baltimore Streetcar Museum.
6. Return to Boy Scout Park.

connecting the walks

Where this walk leaves off you can begin Walk 21: Station North. From Maryland Ave. and Falls Rd., continue straight up W. Lanvale St. to a left on N. Charles St. Pick up the walk from there.

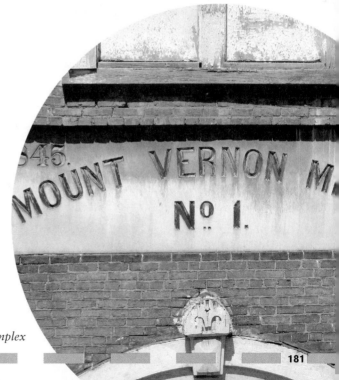

Mount Vernon mill complex

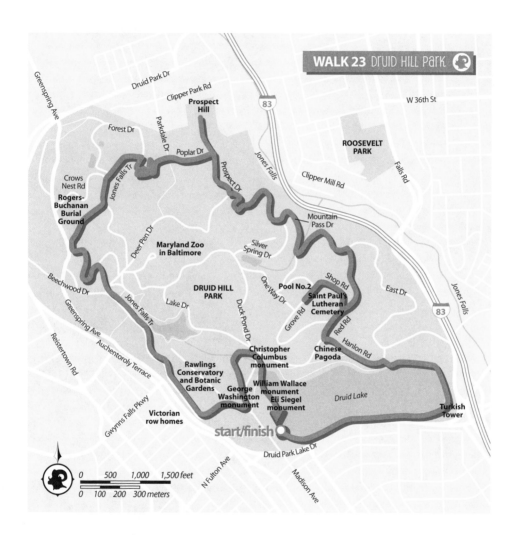

Greenspring Ave

Druid Park Dr

Clipper Park Rd

Prospect Hill

W 36th St

83

Forest Dr

Parkdale Dr

Poplar Dr

Prospect Dr

Jones Falls

ROOSEVELT PARK

Falls Rd

Clipper Mill Rd

Crows Nest Rd

Rogers-Buchanan Burial Ground

Jones Falls Tr

Mountain Pass Dr

Deer Pen Dr

Maryland Zoo in Baltimore

Silver Spring Dr

Beechwood Dr

Jones Falls Tr

Lake Dr

DRUID HILL PARK

One Way Dr

Duck Pond Dr

Pool No.2

Shop Rd

Saint Paul's Lutheran Cemetery

Grove Rd

East Dr

83

Jones Falls

Greenspring Ave

Auchentoroly Terrace

Red Rd

Hanlon Rd

Reisterstown Rd

Rawlings Conservatory and Botanic Gardens

Christopher Columbus monument

Chinese Pagoda

Gwynns Falls Pkwy

George Washington monument

William Wallace monument
Eli Siegel monument

Druid Lake

Turkish Tower

Victorian row homes

start/finish

N Fulton Ave

Druid Park Lake Dr

Madison Ave

0   500   1,000   1,500 feet

0   100   200   300 meters

23 DRUID HILL PARK: THE CITY'S LUNGS

BOUNDARIES: **Druid Park Lake Dr., Greenspring Ave., internal park utility roads (Parkdale Dr., East Dr., Mountain Pass Dr., Prospect Dr., Jones Falls Trail)**

DISTANCE: **4.5 miles**

DIFFICULTY: **Strenuous**

PARKING: **Residential streets ring the park; most allow parking with some restrictions. Additionally, there is abundant parking inside Druid Hill Park.**

PUBLIC TRANSIT: **MTA bus #5 stops at the old Druid Hill Park entrance at Madison Ave. and Druid Lake Park Dr.; MTA bus #53 stops along Auchentoroly Terr.**

Druid Hill Park, a massive urban oasis at 745 acres, was founded in 1860 and created from revenue collected from a penny tax on nickel horsecar fares. In the United States, only Philadelphia's Fairmount and New York's Central rank as older urban landscaped parks. Indeed, it was the Olmsted brothers, fresh off their design of Central Park, who turned their attention to Druid Hill. Despite the great attention to landscape details, whole swaths of the park have been left blissfully alone and now constitute some of the largest intact areas of old-growth forest in Maryland. Druid Hill was originally part of George Buchanan's rolling country estate, and his gorgeous mansion now serves as the Maryland Zoo's administrative home. Druid Hill Park houses not only the state's oldest zoo, but also a whole host of historic sites and buildings, miles of meandering trails (including a lovely portion of the Jones Falls Trail), a public pool, basketball and tennis courts, lots of fun events sponsored by the Friends of Druid Hill (druidhillpark.org) such as annual winter solstice parties, and Druid Park Lake, a magnet for recreation-seekers from all over the city. For those who normally stick to the most developed sections of the park, the rest can be a revelation. Old carriage and bridle paths, once open to automobile traffic, have reverted to pedestrian and bicycle traffic only. A stroll through all four corners of this wonderful park never fails to yield surprises and delights. Baltimore author Upton Sinclair, most famous for his novel *The Jungle,* spent many hours here, later reminiscing, "[Druid Hill] is such a beautiful park. I used to walk over from Grandfather Harden's house on Maryland Avenue with a book of Shakespeare under my arm." That's still a lovely way to spend a day.

● **Begin at the Druid Lake Loop, easily reached from Druid Park Lake Dr. and Madison Ave. Look across Druid Park Lake Dr. along Madison Ave. and Cloverdale Rd. south** and you'll see the impressive stone archway that originally marked the entrance to Druid Hill Park. The archway includes this inscription: "Druid Hill Park. Thomas Swann, Mayor. Inaugurated, 1860." A trolley, part of the long-gone Druid Hill Railway, once stopped here at what used to be wrought iron gates instead of the busy flow of traffic here now. Druid Lake is rather attractive and its 1-mile loop is a popular place for city residents to get some exercise. On your way around, look for two amazing sculptures, hewn by chainsaw from the stumps of dead red oaks. One is *The Druid,* a bearded bust standing 10 feet high. The other is *Green Man,* a nature beast emerging from a den of leaves and vines. The lake, which is ringed with aquatic plants, provides a home to a multitude of ducks, geese, and red-winged blackbirds. In the 19th and early 20th centuries, people headed out onto the lake in rowboats. A lot has changed since those days, but the lake remains just as lovely and is still used for city drinking water. The fountain that sat dormant for more than 10 years was restored to working order in 2004, and multicolored lights below the surface now accompany its nightly sprays. On the southeast corner of Druid Lake is the enigmatic Moorish or Turkish Tower, a squat, white marble structure with club-shaped windows. From here you can see Wyman Park, the bell tower of Gilman Hall on the Johns Hopkins University campus, and the old brick Stieff Silver building, among other notable landmarks. In late March and early April, the hill below is completely covered in yellow tulips.

When you reach the northwestern edge of the lake, look for the little paved path that connects you to Red Rd. and take it heading north. (My recommendation is to first take a few extra steps to Hanlon Dr., which connects to Red Rd., and check out the Chinese Pagoda [1865], a beautiful, multicolored celebration in wood. This served as one of Druid Hill's original three trolley stops.) When you reach Shop Rd., to the left, take it and swing around to the little parking area after the road swerves leftward to behold the iron gates of the amazing Saint Paul's Lutheran Cemetery (1854). This cemetery is not well known even to lifelong Baltimore residents. For many years it was overgrown and neglected, and in the mid-1980s the cemetery was terribly vandalized. Many of the graves were tipped over and cracked. Fortunately, in recent years Martini Lutheran Church members have begun painstakingly restoring the cemetery, even setting about fixing cracked graves.

An interesting note about the cemetery: Victoria Atzerodt is buried here. While you might not recognize her name, her son George Atzerodt was one of the Lincoln assassination conspirators; his role was to kill Vice President Andrew Johnson, an act he ultimately never attempted. When Atzerodt was posthumously pardoned by then-President Andrew Johnson, Victoria and John Atzerodt retrieved their son's remains from Washington and brought him to Baltimore. Victoria and George were interred here at Saint Paul's within the family plot of a Gottlieb Taubert (a presumed fictional name).

● Another historic site, albeit of a very different nature, is close by: Continue around Shop Rd. as it becomes Grove Rd., where you will see tennis courts. This entire area was once known as Druid Hill Park's Negro Section, where African American tennis greats such as Arthur Ashe and Althea Gibson played. To your right is another eerie testament to racial inequality. This rectangular monument filled with dirt and grass is the old Pool No. 2, the 1921 pool restricted to African Americans. The pool, 105 feet by 100 feet (with a paltry deep end of only 7.5 feet), saw between 600 and 1,200 visitors a day during the summers. The lifeguard chairs and ladders are still there now, standing silent witness to pleasant memories managed under the most trying social circumstances.

● Return to Red Rd. (you can go between the tennis courts on the outside of Saint Paul's Cemetery) and go left. At the next three-way intersection, head left, onto East Dr. (These are narrow lanes, closed to automobile traffic and heavily wooded. Often there are no street signs to guide the way.) East Dr. follows a looping route through very thick and picturesque hardwood forest with some particularly lovely sections crowded with mature tulip, oak, poplar, and maple. When East Dr. meets another road (Blacksmith Rd.), head right to stay on East Dr.

The Rawlings Conservatory

Back Story

Near the Rawlings Conservatory used to stand clay tennis courts for white use only. Those courts mark the place where, in 1948, two dozen African Americans and seven white Young Progressives played an integrated match, making it one of the country's first public demonstrations against segregation. It's a shame that so few people, inside Baltimore or out, know this history. Some 500 people showed up to watch, and eventually the police broke it up. H. L. Mencken reported that "a gang of so-called progressives, white and black, went to Druid Hill Park to stage an interracial tennis combat, and were collared and jugged by the cops." Most of the protest-ers were charged with disorderly conduct, and seven of the Young Progressives were convicted of conspiracy. Mencken was horrified: "It is astounding to find so much of the spirit of the Georgia Cracker surviving in the Maryland Free State . . . The public parks are supported by the taxpayer, including the colored taxpayer, for the health and pleasure of the whole people. Why should cops be sent into them to separate those people against their will into separate herds? Why should the law set up distinctions and discriminations which the persons directly affected themselves reject?" By 1956, all of the city parks, including Druid Hill, were fully integrated.

and follow it as it loops around to its next intersection, this time with Mountain Pass Dr. (Again, don't expect trafficked roads here, but rather somewhat desolate blacktop winding through the sort of forest that you'd be forgiven for believing was nowhere near the center of a major populated city. If you're up for some off-trail poking around, there is a surprise around almost every corner. There are stone remains of defunct buildings scattered throughout the woods of the park, many part of the original Buchanan-Rogers estate.)

- Take a right onto Mountain Pass Dr. When it emerges from the woods and links up with Prospect Dr., take a right. Take Prospect Dr. as it once again plunges into deep woods. Pass the next intersection (Poplar Dr.) and continue straight to emerge onto Prospect Hill. This spot was a favorite of Victorian visitors to the park; many late-19th-century prints and postcards depict the view of Woodberry from Prospect Hill. When you've taken it in, return the way you came, but this time take a right onto Poplar Dr. and follow it as it crosses Parkdale Dr. and links up with and becomes the Jones Falls Trail (JFT). (If you're hungry, one of the city's terrific restaurants, Woodberry Kitchen, is just up the trail in Woodberry; see "Connecting the Walks" on page 189.) When complete, the JFT will stretch 12 miles from the Inner Harbor in the south all the way to Robert E. Lee Park just over the city line in Baltimore County, more or less following the course of the Jones Falls. As of this writing, Phases I and III of the trail are complete, with Phase II well on its way.

- The JFT becomes a series of switchbacks built to meet accessibility standards for people in wheelchairs. It's an impressive display and beautifully constructed. Follow the JFT (prominent signage will point the way). You'll soon come to the outer edges of a disc golf course, one of the more popular in the metro area. Be sure to watch out for errant discs. The JFT swings close to Greenspring Ave. before making a U-turn back into the deep woods. As you approach Greenspring Ave., look to the right within a copse of trees (and Hole #2 on the disc golf course) to find the Rogers-Buchanan Burial Ground, founded in the 1700s. It contains grave markers from the 18th century, culminating in Edmund Law Rogers's interment in 1896.

- Continue along the JFT and look for an old circular stone shelter on the right. Follow the JFT as it skirts the edge of a bus parking lot for the Maryland Zoo. The trail then swings around near the entrance to the zoo. Known until recently as the Baltimore Zoo, the Maryland Zoo in Baltimore is the country's third oldest, here since 1876. Attractions include a feeding area for the reticulated giraffes (it's pretty wild experiencing those impossibly long tongues taking the feed from your hands). In 2008, "little" Samson was born, marking the zoo's first elephant birth; the next year, one of the zoo's resident polar bears won a national contest, sponsored by Microsoft, to become the country's best zoo animal. In all, there are more than 2,000 animals on display at the zoo (including my absolute favorite, the beautifully weird-looking okapi).

- Continue along the JFT until you soon reach the stunning Rawlings Conservatory and Botanic Gardens. The Conservatory is one of the city's better-kept secrets; an 1888 glass pavilion serves as the main building, but two new pavilions added in 2004 make this an even more wonderful attraction, offering a chance to see exotic plants and flowers. The main palm building is 50 feet high and sports some 175 windows.

The adjacent orchid room is much smaller in scale, but all those orchids in one place create a pretty spectacular setting as well. In the outside gardens, to the right of the conservatory entrance, you'll find an unusual 1892 sundial, created by stonecutter Peter Hamilton. This spherical, tetradecagon (14-sided) hunk of granite looks like a meteorite. It tells the time for Baltimore, Calcutta, Cape Cod, Cape Town, Fernando Po, Honolulu, Jeddo, Jerusalem, London, Pitcairn Island, Rio de Janeiro, San Francisco, and Sitka. (In 1993, the sundial received some corrections, as it wasn't accurate.)

Look across Greenspring Ave. for the row of arresting Victorian row homes that line the oddly named Auchentoroly (ohk-en-TROLL-ee) Terrace. This row of houses was built between 1876 and the mid-1920s. In the 1720s, this entire area, including part of today's Druid Hill Park, belonged to the Scot George Buchanan, who named his estate Auchentorolie after his ancestral Scottish home. The mansion at 3436 Auchentoroly Terr. was once the home of the Park School (now on a beautiful country spread in Baltimore County), one of the first schools in the city to integrate Jewish and Christian students. The name Druid Hill came later, thought to be inspired by the land's massive oaks and the Druids' love of the trees.

● Baltimore has had many nicknames over the years, including Mobtown for the city's early inhabitants' penchant for fomenting mobs; Charm City, the current nickname; and Monument City, a popular name in the 19th and early 20th centuries for the city's profusion of monuments. Name the person, and there is probably a monument some-where to him or her in Baltimore, as you'll glean from these pages. As you begin to make your way toward Druid Lake on the JFT from the conservatory, you'll see four of these monuments in quick succession, and their eclectic nature truly is a testament to Baltimore's love of monuments. First, look for a memorial to George Washington. It will be facing away from you, but you will see "Presented by the family of Noah Walker" etched in the back. When you reach this, make a U-turn left and follow the path to the lake loop. Head right, passing the small marble monument to Christopher Columbus, copied from a similar statue in Genoa. The simple inscription etched in the marble reads: "Cristoforo Columbo. The Italians of Baltimore, 1892." For years, this statue was a focal point for Italian American celebrations. Continuing around the lake, next up is an impressive statue of a man in chain mail, shield by his side, sword raised above his head; this is William Wallace, Guardian of Scotland. He stands atop five massive granite boulders. William Wallace Spence originally presented the statue on November 30, 1893, and it was rededicated on August 22, 1993, by Baltimore's Society of St. Andrew. Last is Eli Siegel, founder of aesthetic realism; he was born in Latvia but grew up in Baltimore. His likeness is cast onto a bronze plate set into a large rock. You are now where you began.

POINTS OF INTEREST (START TO FINISH)

Moorish Tower Druid Hill Park

Saint Paul's Lutheran Cemetery Druid Hill Park

Pool No. 2 Monument Druid Hill Park

Maryland Zoo in Baltimore marylandzoo.org, Druid Hill Park, 410-396-7102

Rawlings Conservatory rawlingsconservatory.org, 3100 Swann Dr., 410-396-0008

ROUTE SUMMARY

1. Start at the Druid Lake Loop and circle the lake.
2. Use the pedestrian pathway to link up with Red Rd. and turn right.
3. Turn left on Shop Rd. to visit Saint Paul's Lutheran Cemetery and Pool No. 2.
4. Return to Red Rd. and go left.
5. Turn left onto East Dr.
6. Turn right onto Mountain Pass Dr.
7. Turn right onto Prospect Dr.
8. Link with the Jones Falls Trail.
9. Follow the Jones Falls Trail back to Druid Lake.

CONNECTING THE WALKS

Reach Walk 28: Woodberry by taking Parkdale Dr. right from Poplar Dr. instead of linking up with the Jones Falls Trail.

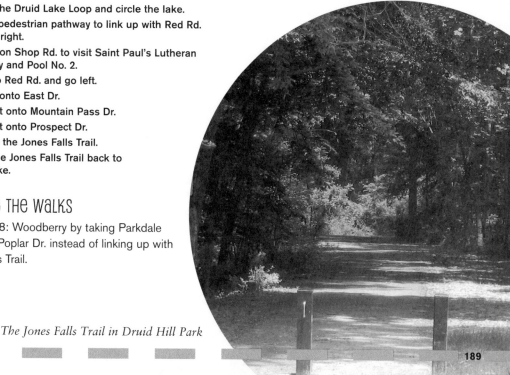

The Jones Falls Trail in Druid Hill Park

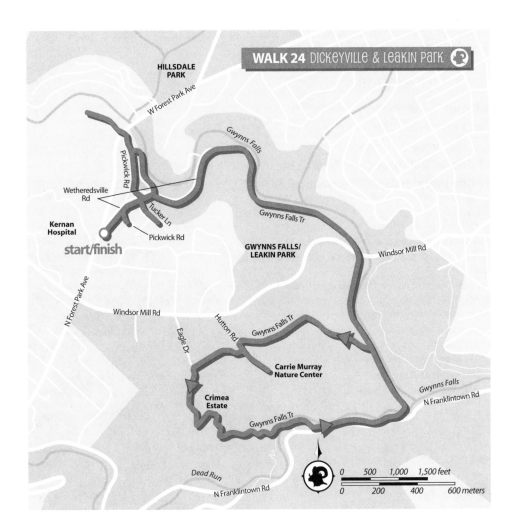

HILLSDALE
PARK

W Forest Park Ave

Gwynns Falls

Pickwick Rd

Wetheredsville
Rd

Tucker Ln

Kernan
Hospital

start/finish

Pickwick Rd

Gwynns Falls Tr

GWYNNS FALLS/
LEAKIN PARK

Windsor Mill Rd

N Forest Park Ave

Windsor Mill Rd

Hutton Rd

Eagle Dr

Gwynns Falls Tr

Carrie Murray
Nature Center

Crimea
Estate

Gwynns Falls Tr

Gwynns Falls

N Franklintown Rd

Dead Run

N Franklintown Rd

0   500   1,000   1,500 feet

0   200   400   600 meters

24 DICKEYVILLE & LEAKIN PARK: MORE CHARM THAN YOU CAN SHAKE A FOREST AT

BOUNDARIES: **N. Forest Park Ave., Pickwick Rd., Wetheredsville Rd., Gwynns Falls Trail/Leakin Park trails**

DISTANCE: **1.5 miles in Dickeyville; 7 miles with Leakin Park add-on**

DIFFICULTY: **Easy in Dickeyville; strenuous with Leakin Park add-on**

PARKING: **Street parking in Dickeyville**

PUBLIC TRANSIT: **MTA bus #15 stops on N. Forest Park Ave., just before Wetheredsville Rd.**

It's a cliché, but there's really little other way to state it: turning off Forest Park Ave. into the enclave of Dickeyville is like performing time travel. There's a reason exploring Dickeyville feels like stepping back in time; Dickeyville's beginnings date to a time when the United States of America was still but a notion. As early as the 1670s, Richard Gwynn set up a post here to trade with native Algonquians. By 1719, the first of what would later become a host of mills popped up on the banks of the Gwynns Falls. The establishment of the village you see today dates to the 1770s. It began to prosper with the building of the Franklin Paper Mill in the early 1800s. Three brothers of the Wethered family converted the mill in 1829 to a woolen mill. The brothers built some 30 stone houses for mill workers, plus a church and a school, and named the village Wetheredsville. In the 1870s, the Wethereds sold the entire area to William Dickey: 300 acres, the mill, and all the surrounding buildings. Dickey died in 1896, but two years later, the village was renamed in his honor. Today, all of Dickeyville is on the National Register of Historic Places. Many original buildings remain, some more than 200 years old and still privately inhabited. Nationally recognized author Laura Lippman, a former *Baltimore Sun* journalist and creator of the popular Tess Monaghan mystery series (among other notable works), grew up in Dickeyville; her 2011 novel, *The Most Dangerous Thing*, is set here, opening with a group of children playing kickball next to a cotton mill on Wetheredsville Road. Lippman consistently proves a great read (she's received effusive praise from notable authors such as Stephen King and Dennis Lehane), but after taking this walk, you'll definitely want to read *The Most Dangerous Thing* if you haven't already—Dickeyville and Leakin Park play the roles of outsize characters, informing the novel's major plot points.

Note: as you wander this lovely village, keep in mind that the houses pointed out below are private residences and should be respected as such.

- From Forest Park Ave., your first right into Dickeyville proper is on Wetheredsville Rd., and the charm of the place hits you immediately with beautiful houses and an abundance of stone: stone gutters, stone driveways, roadside stone walls. Dickeyville residents labor over beautification projects, which still mark this lovely little village—note the Belgian block and stone lining the streets. The red house to your right, at 5131 Wetheredsville, was built around 1850 and was once the home of Billy Ware, a soldier in the Union Army who served as a flag-bearer at the Battle of Gettysburg.

- Continue on Wetheredsville Rd. The extraordinary stone beauty with the red shutters at 5123 Wetheredsville was built around 1810 and belonged to Amos Humphries, one of the founders of the Independent Order of Odd Fellows. Soon after is the 1885 white clapboard Dickey Memorial Presbyterian Church. The house next door, 5116 Wetheredsville, was the minister's house, which dates to 1890. Across the street, the white house (circa 1840) was once the home of the Ashland Mill's manager. Soon after is the intersection of Wetheredsville and Pickwick Rd. Nearby notable homes include #5104 and #5106, both built circa 1840. The brick duplex at #5100 dates to 1854.

- Take a right up Pickwick Rd. Pickwick was not the original name of this street. Originally, Hillsworth, Forest, and Main Sts. ran through here, but early residents, in their desire to have their town resemble an English country village (thus the preponderance of stone), chose Pickwick to better fit their vision. You can see the original stone springhouse (circa 1853) at 2309 Pickwick. Built in 1900, #2305 was originally a carriage house.

- Return to Wetheredsville Rd. and take a right. The house at 5107 Wetheredsville was built circa 1810 by Elias Reed, who owned the nearby Wakefield Plantation (no longer in existence). A few decades later, the village lamplighter, Frank Page, lived in this house. Nearby is #5101. It was built as the Mechanics Institute in the 1890s and functioned as a lodge for the Junior Order of American Mechanics. A concert hall inside used to host vaudeville and minstrel shows.

- The small intersecting street to the right is Tucker Ln. Take a quick right up here to see a series of 19th-century houses lining the left side of the street. The oldest of them dates to 1825 and is at #2317. The man who gave his name to the street lived in the circa 1881 house at #2300 at the top of the hill.

- Return to Wetheredsville Rd. and take a right. Next up, on the left, is the gorgeous stone Ashland Chapel (its physical address is actually on Pickwick). It's now a private residence, but it was originally built in 1849 as a Quaker Meeting House. As you approach another intersection (Wetheredsville and Wetheredsville, believe it or not), you'll see at the edge of the Ashland Chapel property a little conical shed that once served as a trolley stop.

- Take a left so that the chapel is on your left, passing three houses on your right, and link up with Pickwick Rd. Take a right onto Pickwick. Close by, at 2322 Pickwick, was the home of another village shopkeeper. The arresting Victorian Gothic at 2332 Pickwick (circa 1832) was apparently an officers' quarters originally built at Fort McHenry before being moved here; the steep pitch of the roofs was included to encourage artillery to roll off. #2326 and #2330 were built circa 1875; #2322 predates them, circa 1835.

- Continuing on Pickwick, you'll soon come to what many consider to be the most visually interesting block in Dickeyville, anchored by the extraordinary four-story stone buildings at 2407 and 2411 Pickwick. The buildings predate the Civil War and housed mill families. Both are visually arresting with patterned brick interrupting the excellent stonework around each arched window. Take notice of the gas lamp at #2407; it's a replica of one at Philadelphia's Independence Hall. Next door, #2405, built at the same time, used to function as a village store owned by William Dickey, and once housed the YWCA.

  Other nearby buildings on Pickwick include: #2412, which was constructed in 1853 and functioned as an

Typical Dickeyville architecture

Independent Order of Odd Fellows lodge. After its original purpose, it enjoyed life as a general store, with a gas station out front and post office inside. The extension on the house was once a pharmacy. #2415 and #2417 date to circa 1870–75.

The extraordinary stone and brick General Grant building at 2423 Pickwick was built in 1872. Baltimore artist R. McGill Mackall used the house as a studio. Mackall was born in Baltimore in 1899 and studied not only in Baltimore and New York, but also at the Royal Institute of Art in Munich and the Academie Julian in Paris. After returning to Baltimore, he painted 53 large murals that graced various locations in the city, almost half of which still survive. His largest mural measures 14 by 80 feet and stands in the Great Hall of the War Memorial building downtown (see Walk 12: Downtown: Contrasts). During his career, he served as head of the fine arts department at MICA and founded the art department at the College of Notre Dame of Maryland. (For what it's worth, author Lippman remembered Mackall as something of a crank, perpetually shooing neighborhood kids off his back lawn.)

● Continue north on Pickwick. #2418–2430 all date from 1875 and are good examples of Dickeyville's mill housing. Built in 1832, 2432 Pickwick is an Early Republic house. The home at #2433 (circa 1875) once belonged to Malcolm Moos, an advisor to President Dwight Eisenhower, and was outfitted with a direct telephone connection to the White House. Nearby, #2435 was once a mill office, built in 1840. A first-floor room also held the occasional criminal, serving as an overflow for the jail. President Teddy Roosevelt once gave an impromptu speech here. As you continue up Pickwick, the houses become more modern, but no less lovely. Follow Pickwick to its intersection with N. Forest Park Ave. To your left, at the intersection, you'll see a sign: "Dickeyville: Founded 1772, Restored 1934."

● Cross N. Forest Park Ave. by staying on Pickwick. (Take some caution here; it's a sometimes-busy road with a blind curve.) Immediately to the left, up the hill, you'll see the impressive house at #2500. Local historians date this house to 1790, and many believe it began as an Indian Trading Post. Its proximity to the Gwynns Falls, just to your right, would support this. The house later served as housing for mill workers. Pickwick carries on for another few hundred feet before stopping abruptly in the forested flanks of the northwest edges of Leakin Park. Most of the houses on the left side of the street are more modern, while those on the right side mostly date to the 1870s. The village magistrate lived at #2515, built in 1875. #2541 was known locally as the Wagon Wheel House for the large wagon wheel embedded into one of the house's walls.

● Turn around here and retrace your route back across N. Forest Park Ave. When you reach the stone house at #2435, take a left down the little path between houses toward the water. (If you aren't up for any hiking, skip the next six bullet points and proceed to Wetheredsville Rd. If you want to extend this walk into the beauty of Leakin Park and check out more historic sites in the park, follow the next six bullet points. But be aware: it makes of this walk a hike, but one well worth your time.)

● The path, here called Cottondale Ln., runs behind the houses on Pickwick, flanking the Gwynns Falls. You'll see a dam in the water, which was built after Hurricane Agnes washed away the original wooden dam in 1972. Just upstream, on the northern bank, is where the original Franklin Paper Mill stood (built in 1800 and destroyed by fire in 1934). As you approach Wetheredsville Rd. again, stick to the little path that parallels the water. Soon, you'll pop out of the woods momentarily as you rejoin Wetheredsville, here closed to vehicle traffic and serving as part of the Gwynns Falls Trail (GFT).

● Follow the paved GFT through thick urban forest. This forest, spanning Gwynns Falls and Leakin Parks, constitutes one of the largest unbroken urban forests in the United States. Leakin Park itself is larger than New York's Central Park and remains one of the city's greatest, if underappreciated, gems. It's spectacular, with much soaring second-growth forest. If you were dropped here from a plane, you would never guess you were in the middle of an industrialized city; all you can see are sky and trees. Portions of the hit movie *The Blair Witch Project* were shot here, and the thick forest makes it easy to see why. You'll eventually approach Windsor Mill Rd., which you should cross, staying on the GFT on the other side. When you reach an intersection, take a right onto the old Hutton Rd., here closed to vehicle traffic.

● Follow Hutton Rd. until another intersection, this one Ridgetop Rd., and take a left to reach the Carrie Murray Nature Center. As you walk this short stretch of paved road, note the little path on your right opposite the small parking area to your left; you'll return this way.

The nature center was named for the mother of Orioles Hall of Famer Eddie Murray. Most interesting is the rehabilitation center for injured birds of prey; the center also provides a nice display of reptiles.

● Moving away from the nature center, turn back toward the small parking area and take the little path noted above, now to your left. You'll see white blazes on this trail, which is very dense and well shaded, mostly by tall oaks, and again you'll feel as if you can't possibly be anywhere near Baltimore. The blazes soon turn red, and you'll see a sign pointing to the Ridge Trail, but go straight. To the left you'll see pavilions, picnic benches, a parking area, playground, volleyball net, and tennis courts. You'll also see a boarded-up chapel to the left; colorful wildflowers surround it in spring and summer. When the trail emerges from the woods onto a paved road (Eagle Dr.) and parking lot, turn left. To your right you'll see train tracks through the open field; these belong to the Chesapeake & Allegheny Steam Preservation Society Headquarters, which was constructed to look like an old train depot. The Chesapeake & Allegheny Live Steamers, a miniature steam-powered railroad with 3,400 feet of track, offers free rides every second Sunday of the month, April through November.

● Take the paved Eagle Dr. toward the woods. You'll soon pass several stone buildings on your right and will ultimately see the carriage house, chapel, caretaker's house, and honeymoon cottage of the Crimea Estate. Pass the headquarters of the Baltimore Chesapeake Bay Outward Bound and end up at the spectacular Orianda House at the end of the loop. Orianda was built in 1856–57 as a summer retreat by Thomas Winans, who made a fortune in Russia overseeing construction of the transcontinental railroad for Czar Nicholas I. He called the estate Crimea after the Russian peninsula of the same name. The owners, who were known Southern-sympathizers, tried to discourage Union troops from entering their estate during the Civil War by constructing a faux fort with fake cannons. It didn't work; the troops of General Benjamin Butler cut up the orchard for firewood, arrested Winans's father Ross, and locked him away in Fort McHenry.

● You have a couple of options at this point. The quickest and easiest route back to your starting point is to head back north on Eagle Dr. to Windsor Mill Rd. and take a right to the point you passed earlier on the GFT; however, Windsor Mill is a busy road and the sidewalk gives out, making this a potentially dangerous option. Alternately, you can retrace your steps along the GFT you took to get here from Dickeyville. Another option takes you a bit deeper into Leakin Park, but does extend this hike a few miles. If you are up for it, head downhill from the Orianda House into the woods. Be careful—the trail is rocky here, and it's easy to twist a knee. After about a hundred yards, you'll see a foot trail to the right; follow it through a magnificent stand of white oaks. The trail gets a little tighter here in summertime, and a few sections are washed away from erosion, but this is a relatively short section. Soon, when you come to a T intersection, head left. You'll arrive in a big clearing with picnic benches and a pavilion, the Ben Cardin picnic grove, named after the Baltimore congressman and Maryland senator. Walk downhill toward the patch of wetlands next to the pavilion. Walk along the paved path and cross over Dead Run on the bridge to the parking area at Winans Meadow, a central location for visitors arriving at Leakin Park. Head right on the paved path at the parking area. When you see a footbridge over Dead Run to the left, pass it and cross over on a pretty steel bridge. Immediately to the left is Wetheredsville Rd. again, here closed to traffic. This is the same Wetheredsville Rd. you were on before, but just in a different spot. You can follow it all the way back to Dickeyville.

● Returning to Dickeyville: When you passed this way before, heading into Leakin Park, you bypassed this section of Wetheredsville Rd. Now, as you emerge from the GFT, you'll see the nearby houses on Wetheredsville. Of note is #4901, the first house you'll pass. This house was built in 1865 for John Melville, the superintendent of the Ashland Mill. Look for the small building to the left of the main residence; this is the original springhouse. Martin Tshudi, who built the first mill in 1762, originally lived in this location; while his home no longer exists, the gravestones of his wife and daughter

Welcome to Dickeyville

are still close by. Across from #4901 is the location of the old Ashland Mill. Also built in 1865, #5008 sits astride the 1830 rubblestone structure at #5002, which originally served as the Dickeyville school. #5009 was constructed in 1890. #5010 was built in 1910 and served originally as the home of the Cherry Cough Syrup Company and later became a tavern and then a garage. #5012 was built in 1840 and served as a free dispensary; #5016 was built in 1840 for Charles Wethered, one of the three brothers of the mill-owning family; the open area across from #5017 was once a trolley stop, running the line from Lorraine Cemetery to Walbrook Junction. You can still see the original rails in the road.

● A bit farther up the road, the gorgeous house at #5023 was built in 1835 and served various incarnations, including village apothecary and a candy store. You'll see two smaller houses flanking this one; the candy store owner built these for his sons as they married. The house next door, at #5027, often stops people. It was built in the 1940s and was designed to mimic George Washington's Mount Vernon and is known locally as Little Mount Vernon. The house at #5029 (circa 1850) served as the home of the village dairy cow (that's right) and then later became a glove factory. Soon, you will pass Pickwick again, and soon after that will be your starting point—a long, but most probably satisfying day.

POINTS OF INTEREST (START TO FINISH)

For Dickeyville, see text for specific sites. For more information on Dickeyville, visit dickeyville.org

For Leakin Park:

Carrie Murray Nature Center carriemurraynaturecenter.org, 1901 Ridgetop Rd., 410-396-0808

Chesapeake & Allegheny Steam Preservation Society Headquarters (Chesapeake & Allegheny Live Steamers) calslivesteam.org, 4921 Windsor Mill Rd., 410-448-0730

Orianda House/Crimea Estate friendsoforiandahouse.com, Leakin Park, 1901 Eagle Dr., 410-299-7613

friendsofgwynnsfallsleakinpark.org

route summary

1. Start at Wetheredsville Rd., just off N. Forest Park Ave.

2. Turn right on Pickwick Rd.

3. Return to Wetheredsville Rd. and take a right.

4. Take a right onto Tucker Ln.

5. Return to Wetheredsville Rd and take a right.

6. Take a left past the Ashland Chapel and then a right onto Pickwick Rd.

7. Cross N. Forest Park Ave. to the end of Pickwick Rd. and then return on Pickwick Rd.

8. Take a left onto Cottondale Ln. and link up with the Gwynns Falls Trail. (If not hiking in Leakin Park, skip the rest of the directions and return to your starting point on Wetheredsville Rd. If hiking in Leakin Park, go to #9.)

9. Take the GFT into Leakin Park across Windsor Mill Rd.

10. Take a right onto Hutton Rd.

11. Take a left onto Ridgetop Rd. to the Carrie Murray Nature Center.

12. Take the dirt path north of the nature center left to paved Eagle Dr.

13. Turn left onto Eagle Dr. and follow it to the Orianda House/Crimea Estate.

14. Take the dirt path down the hill from Orianda to the Ben Cardin Picnic Grove and Winans Meadow trailhead and parking lot in Leakin Park.

15. Head east on the paved path and cross Dead Run.

16. Take a left onto Wetheredsville Rd. and follow it back to Dickeyville.

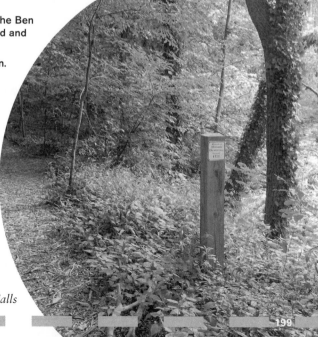

Wooded trail along the Gwynns Falls

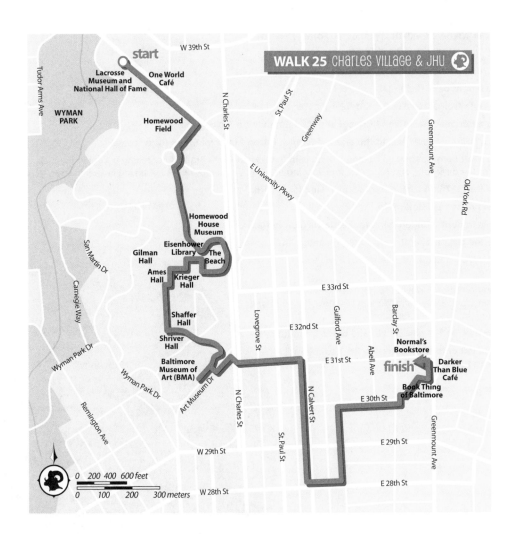

start

W 39th St

Lacrosse
Museum and
National Hall of Fame

One World
Café

Tudor Arms Ave

WYMAN
PARK

Homewood
Field

N Charles St

St. Paul St

Greenway

E University Pkwy

Greenmount Ave

Old York Rd

San Martin Dr

Homewood
House
Museum

Eisenhower
Library

Gilman
Hall

The
Beach

Ames
Hall

Krieger
Hall

E 33rd St

Carnegie Way

Shaffer
Hall

Guilford Ave

Barclay St

Shriver
Hall

Lovegrove St

E 32nd St

Normal's
Bookstore

Wyman Park Dr

Baltimore
Museum of
Art (BMA)

E 31st St

Abell Ave

finish

Darker
Than Blue
Café

Wyman Park Dr

Art Museum Dr

N Charles St

N Calvert St

E 30th St

Book Thing
of Baltimore

Remington Ave

St. Paul St

E 29th St

Greenmount Ave

W 29th St

E 28th St

0   200 400 600 feet

0   100   200   300 meters

W 28th St

25 Charles Village & JHU: Baltimore's Image Builder

BOUNDARIES: **W. University Pkwy., Johns Hopkins University Homewood Campus, E. 28th St., Greenmount Ave.**

DISTANCE: **3 miles**

DIFFICULTY: **Moderate**

PARKING: **Street parking, with some residential restrictions, all along route**

PUBLIC TRANSIT: **MTA buses #22 and #61 stop along University Pkwy. at JHU. MTA bus #11 runs north–south along N. Charles St., stopping at JHU. MTA bus #3 stops in Charles Village. MTA bus #8 runs north–south along Greenmount Ave. and stops near the Darker Than Blue Café.**

In recent decades, Baltimore has suffered an image problem. While Baltimore spent much of America's early years as a center of commerce and industry and one of the nation's largest and most important cities, its decline in the 20th century due to dwindling manufacturing jobs and flight to the suburbs meant that Baltimore, like many Rust Belt cities, was guaranteed some hard times. Even in the face of the urban renaissance of the 1980s–2000s, most people around the country know Baltimore primarily as one of the country's most dangerous cities, consistently ranking near the top of national statistics for murders per capita and violent crime. Through the first decades of the new millennium, these numbers have been declining, but popular television shows such as *Homicide: Life on the Street* and *The Wire* presented the country with fresh imagery of Baltimore as a crime-riddled cesspool. Of course, those of us who live here know better. But tenacious pockets of crime and poverty still persist and, as we know, perception is sometimes everything. Good thing, then, for Baltimore that it can also claim some world-class institutions. The Johns Hopkins University & Hospital, the federal government's top private research institution and the country's first research university, top the list. The hospital's annual ranking as the best in the country is routine, and its presence, along with all the adjuncts the university and hospital spawn, assure that Baltimore will forever also be associated with something great. This walk begins at the campus of the vaunted university—home to a bevy of Nobel laureates (36 at last count)—and takes in the surrounding neighborhood of Charles Village, known for its diversity and tolerance.

● Start at the Lacrosse Museum and National Hall of Fame at 113 W. University Pkwy., adjacent to the Johns Hopkins University. The museum covers this fast-growing sport that has always found a hotbed in Baltimore, spanning from the game's American Indian roots all the way to the present. Its location next to JHU makes sense: the men's team has won nine national championships since 1970. Continuing east on W. University Pkwy., you'll pass Homewood Field, the home field of all those great teams. If you're looking for good vegan eats and a popular local hangout, try One World Café, across the street from Homewood at 100 W. University. You might just run into actor and frequent visitor John Astin, Hopkins grad and theater professor, best known for his Edgar Allan Poe one-man shows/impersonations and, of course, for the lead of Gomez Addams in the popular 1960s television sitcom *The Addams Family*.

● When you've passed Homewood Field, take a right onto the JHU campus, taking the path between Homewood Field and the baseball diamond. When Johns Hopkins died the day before Christmas, 1873, he left behind $7 million for the founding of a university and a hospital—the largest bequest in the history of the country at the time. He had amassed considerable wealth as an investor and later as director of the B&O Railroad and he had no heirs. Construction on both the university and the hospital began almost immediately, but the university's location at its present site at Homewood didn't begin until 1902. The university set up an architectural advisory board that year, and it included the venerable Frederick Law Olmsted Jr. It was another decade before construction could begin—with proceeds from sales of Hopkins's buildings, grants from the state, and money from a Rockefeller philanthropic organization. By 1915, Gilman and Maryland Halls were complete.

JHU's campus is a beautiful one, with Georgian- and Federal-style architecture designed to mimic that of the oldest building on campus, the Homewood House. You'll be there shortly, but for now, head left when you reach the parking circle in front of the Athletic Center. I encourage you to wander all around the lovely campus. It feels older than its 100 years and would fit in just fine with the Ivy League's older institutions. (Indeed, it stood in for Harvard in the 2011 film *The Social Network*.) But to hit the highlights, continue along the path, passing dorms to your left, and through the Freshman Quad, until you come directly to the Eisenhower Library. To the left, beyond the trees, is the Homewood House Museum. Built in 1801, the house originally belonged to the family of Charles Carroll, signer of the Declaration of

Independence. It has been the property of JHU since 1902 and has been listed on the National Register of Historic Places since 1971. Today, it serves as a public museum, showcasing 19th-century artifacts and re-creating early 19th-century life in Baltimore.

The entrance to Homewood House looks out over the ellipse of The Beach, the circular green space fronting N. Charles St., where the campus has slipped its original borders and spilled over into Charles Village. At the bottom of The Beach is the East Gate, with N. Charles St. just beyond. Directly across from the East Gate, take notice of the building on the south side of E. 34th St. That is JHU's Wolman Hall, an undergraduate residence hall. Wolman Hall used to be the Cambridge Arms Apartments, where F. Scott Fitzgerald lived for several years in the 1930s. His essay "Afternoon of an Author" is a recounting of his battle with writer's block. In the essay, he writes of going to his window and watching "students changing classes on the college campus across the way."

- Go back to the Eisenhower Library and pass it, entering the Keyser Quad, the center of campus. JHU's most notable building is straight ahead: Gilman Hall, unmistakable with its distinctive bell tower. Named for JHU's first president, Daniel Coit Gilman, it was the first major academic building on campus. It recently received an $85 million renovation, which includes a beautiful new museum of archaeology boasting some 8,000 pieces dating from 4,000 B.C. to just a few hundred years ago.

- Leaving Gilman Hall, head back toward the Eisenhower Library, but this time take a right between Ames and Krieger Halls onto the Wyman Quad. When you reach Shriver Hall, straight ahead, go left, passing Shaffer

Charles Village's Painted Ladies

Hall on your left. You'll now be entering the Baltimore Museum of Art's (BMA) outdoor sculpture garden, a wonderful 3-acre space beautifully landscaped and thoughtfully designed to allow private reflection amid the wonderful collection of mostly modernist sculpture spanning the last century.

● Admission to the BMA is free, so definitely take the time to head inside—but not before walking toward Art Museum Dr. to see the building's original grand entrance. It's a classic structure, spectacular in its bold but simple elegance. The acclaimed American architect John Russell Pope designed the building in the 1920s. Its old entrance is notable for the six colossal columns and tapering stone steps. The enormous stone lions flanking the entrance are a nice touch too. This is the museum's original footprint. A huge wing for contemporary art has been part of the museum since 1994. This wing underwent a three-year, $24 million renovation, with significant upgrades and changes, primarily to the museum's American, African, and Contemporary collections. The renovation was completed in fall 2012.

While the Walters Art Museum in Mount Vernon is the city's classical and internationally known jewel, the Baltimore Museum of Art (BMA) is its modern counterpart, with a wonderful collection concentrating on the 20th century. The museum today holds some 90,000 objects; its claim to fame is that it holds the world's largest collection of works by French impressionist Henri Matisse. You'll also find paintings and drawings by Cézanne, Picasso, and van Gogh, among other famous artists. But it's not just the Impressionists who steal the museum's spotlight. There are also other important works in Abstract Expressionism, Minimalism, and Pop Art (with an impressive collection of Warhols). But even though the museum has gained an international reputation as a repository of essential modern works, there are also many terrific prints and paintings dating back to the 15th century, with works by artists such as Botticelli, Sir Anthony van Dyck, and Rembrandt. The first floor houses an extraordinary collection of indigenous art from around the world, including one of the country's most impressive African collections.

● Leave the BMA and head east, crossing N. Charles St. at E. 31st St. There are plenty of eating options here, at Hopkins Square and the surrounding blocks. The area has an energetic feel one would expect so close to a major university. Continue down E. 31st St., and you'll soon be in the heart of Charles Village. The neighborhood dates back to the late 1860s and consists of rows of brownstones and brick row homes, varying in size and complexity of detail. There is an active neighborhood association, and residents take great pride in the high level of diversity and tolerance you'll find here; it has a reputation as something of a bohemian enclave. The neighborhood is home to a large gay and lesbian population, and many Hopkins professors make their homes here. What attracts visitors and tourists to the neighborhood is the Painted Ladies, the many Victorian row houses that have been decked out in bold and often nonmatching colors. Entire façades, porches, doors—everything gets the paint. These houses often grace regional travel guides and export the image of Baltimore as a quirky town. Take time to wander all the streets in Charles Village, but to see the best examples of the Painted Ladies, follow the route here.

- At N. Calvert St., take a right. You'll be heading south. After the next block (E. 30th St.), the houses turn to an impressive collection of large brick homes. You'll notice that the bump-outs above the porches on the right side of the street all sport different paint jobs, an especially interesting effect when two adjoining houses, which share the triangular pitch above their porches, split colors right down the middle. Continue along N. Calvert St. past E. 29th St. for more painted houses—there are more impressive ones to come.

- Take a left onto E. 28th St. and go one block to a left onto Guilford Ave. When you cross E. 30th St., you'll see perhaps the most oft-photographed Painted Ladies. And you'll immediately see why; the crazy quilt of colors—purples, blues, yellows, reds, greens, and pinks—somehow all work in concert to create a wonderful kaleidoscope.

- Return to E. 30th St. and take a right. Follow it two blocks and take a left just after Barclay St. onto Vineyard Ln. Just up to the right is the wonderful Book Thing of Baltimore. If you like books, this is heaven: go inside and take whatever you like—yes, it's all free (but only open on weekends). The Book Thing relies on donations and allows folks to haul off whatever they want—reasonableness and manners are expected, however. This wonderful act of philanthropy has garnered national press, with write-ups in the *New York Times* and *Chicago Tribune,* to name just two outlets.

- Continue on Vineyard Ln. another hundred feet or so until you come to Greenmount Ave. (Old York Rd.). Just up on the left, at 3034 Greenmount Ave., is the Darker Than

Blue Café, a terrific restaurant and cultural hot spot. According to its mission statement, the Darker Than Blue is "rooted in the experience of the African Diaspora and fuses the unique nuances of African American culture with the sophisticated palate of today's discerning diner." To that end, you will find simply terrific food with a Southern flavor (hands down the best corn bread in the city) accompanied by marvelous music. Check out the Sunday jazz brunch for a special treat.

● Go north on Greenmount Ave. (left out of the Darker Than Blue) to the first left onto E. 31st St. Just on your left is Normal's Bookstore. For more than 20 years, Normal's has collected the accolades—it's a consistent Best of Baltimore honoree. You'll find an eclectic and extensive collection of books, records, and CDs here. But what's most special is the unmistakable and irredeemable whiff of anarchy in the place—it's the quintessential Baltimore bookstore in that it celebrates the revolutionary and delightfully off-kilter. It's run by a collective and proudly proclaims: "the collective was involved in a lot of publishing, performance, organizing, alternative thinking, politics, & 'strange' sensibilities . . . The place has always meant more than just selling stuff."

● You can use E. 31st St. to return to JHU (or you can wander a bit more around Charles Village; any of the next four northern blocks will get you there as well— these are E. 32nd St., E. 33rd St., E. 34th St., and University Pkwy.).

POINTS OF INTEREST (START TO FINISH)

Lacrosse Museum and National Hall of Fame uslacrosse.org/museum/halloffame, 113 W. University Pkwy., 410-235-6882

One World Café 100 W. University Pkwy., 410-235-5777

Homewood House Museum (Johns Hopkins University) museums.jhu.edu/homewood, 3400 N. Charles St., 410-516-5589

Gilman Hall (Johns Hopkins University)

The Baltimore Museum of Art artbma.org, 10 Art Museum Dr., 443-573-1700

The Book Thing of Baltimore bookthing.org, 3001 Vineyard Ln., 410-662-5631

Darker Than Blue Café darkerthanbluecafe.com, 3034 Greenmount Ave., 443-872-4468

Normal's Bookstore normals.com, 425 E. 31st St., 410-243-6888

route summary

1. Start at the Lacrosse Museum and National Hall of Fame on W. University Pkwy.
2. Enter Johns Hopkins University Homewood Campus between Homewood Field and the baseball diamond.
3. Pass through the Freshman Quad to the Homewood Museum.
4. Pass through the Keyser Quad to Gilman Hall and the Archaeology Museum.
5. Pass through Wyman Quad to the Baltimore Museum of Art.
6. Cross Art Museum Dr. and N. Charles St. to E. 31st St.
7. Take a right onto N. Calvert St.
8. Take a left onto E. 28th St.
9. Take a left onto Guilford Ave.
10. Visit the 3000 block of Guilford Ave.
11. Take a right onto E. 30th St.
12. Take a left onto Vineyard Ln.
13. Take a left onto Greenmount Ave.
14. Take a left onto E. 31st St.
15. Return to JHU via E. 31st St. or other east–west streets.

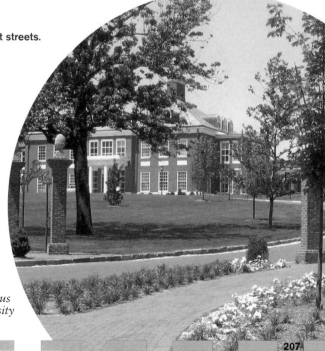

Newer construction on the campus of Johns Hopkins University

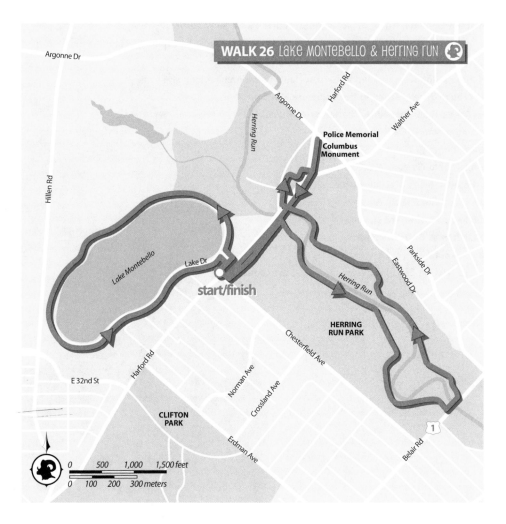

Argonne Dr

Harford Rd

Argonne Dr

Walther Ave

Herring Run

Police Memorial

Columbus Monument

Hillen Rd

Lake Montebello

Lake Dr

Parkside Dr

Eastwood Dr

start/finish

Herring Run

HERRING RUN PARK

Harford Rd

Chesterfield Ave

E 32nd St

Norman Ave

Crossland Ave

CLIFTON PARK

Erdman Ave

Belair Rd

1

0   500   1,000   1,500 feet

0   100   200   300 meters

26 Lake Montebello & Herring Run: Northeast's recreational Havens

BOUNDARIES: **Lake Dr., Herring Run Trail, Belair Rd., Harford Rd.**
DISTANCE: **4.2 miles**
DIFFICULTY: **Moderate**
PARKING: **Parking in designated spaces on lake loop**
PUBLIC TRANSIT: **MTA bus #19 runs along Harford Rd; MTA bus #15 runs along Belair. Rd.**

One of Baltimore's lesser-known attributes (even to many locals) is its preponderance of green spaces. From very early on, city planners recognized the need for Baltimore's citizenry to have access to the country that makes Maryland such an attractive place to live. This mind-set persisted even as the city boomed to become, for several decades in the early and mid-1800s, the country's second largest. Penny and nickel horsecar taxes, a green-minded and progressive citizenry, and the continual employ of the Olmsted brothers, the country's foremost landscape architects, transformed the growing city into a collection of pocketed oases of public parks, lakes, and leafy neighborhoods that worked with the sweeps and curves of the natural landscape. Baltimoreans still enjoy these foresighted results today, and spots like Lake Montebello and Herring Run are just two. The adjacent lakeside neighborhood of Ednor Gardens–Lakeside was once part of the massive estate of Revolutionary War hero and Baltimore Mayor Samuel Smith, who named his manse Montebello after the 1800 battle in Lombardy. Conjoined Herring Run Park snakes for 300 acres through Belair-Edison and is yet another prized recreational haven. The namesake stream needs some further cleaning, but the Herring Run Watershed Association has been and continues to be on the case. On this pleasant walk, join northeast denizens as they take advantage of two of the places that make this part of Baltimore, home to nearby Morgan State University, an underappreciated destination.

● The entrance to the Lake Montebello Lake Loop is just off Harford Rd. (You can take an MTA bus here, or if you drive, enter on Lake Montebello Terr. and head left; there's plenty of parking on the side of the street roughly one quarter of the way around the lake.)

● The route here is obvious; take a stroll around the lake. Lake Montebello is in actuality a large holding tank, fed by Herring Run, before the water is purified for city drinking water. The Lake Montebello Dam was created in 1880; the lake has a surface area of 55 acres (30 feet wide and 600 feet long) and saw a $20 million restoration in 2007. City crews removed sludge buildup and gave the lake new plantings, roadwork, and an iron fence. The city also added a median, complete with flowers and ornamental grasses, which separates cars from the clearly delineated hiking and biking lanes.

● As you walk around the lake, you'll no doubt take notice of what a treasured recreational space this is, with many walkers, strollers, joggers, and bikers. You'll probably also notice the avian life; the red-winged blackbird is prominent here, preferring the tall aquatic grasses near the water's edge. The neighborhood surrounding the lake is known as Mayfield. On the National Register of Historic Places, the neighborhood was built between the late-19th and early to mid-20th centuries (and is home to HBO's *The Wire*'s fictional detective James McNulty).

● If you're interested, when you reach the southwest corner of the lake, just before the leftward exit point on Lake Dr., you can head up the little rise toward E. 33rd St. to see the unmistakable 18-foot statue of Martin Luther looming over the lake, right hand outstretched. The artist was Hans Schuler, a Baltimorean and the first American to win a Salon Gold Medal in Paris. He eventually became director at MICA, serving between 1935 and 1951. This statue dates to 1901.

● When you've made a complete circuit of the lake and find yourself at Lake Montebello Terr., head down to Harford Rd. and cross at the intersection of Montebello Terr., Harford Rd., and Chesterfield Ave., near the Francis of Assisi Church. Once you've crossed, head left down the hill on the paved trail. Hooper Field, ringed by mature trees, opens up to your right. This path continues to descend until Harford Rd. is high above you to the left.

● When you come to the T-intersection, with the Harford Road Bridge to the left, take a right. Herring Run is on your left inside a stand of woods. Soon you'll enter thick forest and come to a little stone bridge. To the right are some beautiful rock formations, creating natural cavelike shelters. Just beyond to the left you'll see a sign informing you that you are in Fox Den. Each subsequent new stretch is named differently, with unobtrusive signs telling you as much. Old oaks and maples dominate this truly magnificent, isolated, idyllic stretch of forest. The trail remains wide and paved, with lots of underbrush and trees towering above on either side. Subsequently, you'll pass through Deep Forest and then Orlinsky Grove. Here the trail follows Herring Run's natural curve and then opens up as a field comes into view on the right. Straight ahead is Belair Rd.; if you head left, you'll see a little dirt path to the water. This is a good place to stand—on either side, the water moves quickly over a series of rocks, while straight ahead it runs smoothly past a nice rock outcrop.

- Use Belair Rd. to cross Herring Run. Once across the Run on Belair, take a left back onto the trail and into the woods. Cross a raised bridge over a small tributary. This section is called Second Tributary, and the path opens up as the trail swings around to the right, passing ball fields to the left. A series of brick duplexes to the right pops up in the clearing up the hill. You'll next come to East Woods Field. Take the paved trail and cross over First Tributary. The path runs much closer to the water on this side than it did on the outbound side. A series of rocks in the water gives off a pleasing sound, almost enough to drown out the sound of traffic, which you'll hear again as soon as you approach Harford Rd. When you reach the bridge, walk under it.

- Once clear of the bridge, take a right onto the little service road and follow it, paralleling Harford Rd. above you to the right. You'll soon see a parking area on your right and a little path leading to Harford Rd. beyond it. Take that and emerge onto the sidewalk on Harford Rd. and take a left, passing Walther Ave.

- Once past Walther Ave., cross Harford Rd. and head into the grassy area, moving to your left toward the tall white obelisk. This unassuming 40-foot piece of public art holds a somewhat amazing distinction: it is the world's oldest standing monument to Christopher Columbus. The story goes that the French Consul to Baltimore, Charles Francois Adrien de Paulmier, was told, as the 300th anniversary of Columbus's voyage to the Americas approached, that there were no monuments to Columbus anywhere in the New World. Seeking to rectify that, the consul had this one built in 1792 and placed it on his estate, originally near where North Ave. and Harford Rd. meet. The statue stood there until 1964, when it was moved to its present site.

- Just a couple of hundred feet away is another memorial, this one more poignant than celebratory, at the corner of Harford Rd. and Parkside Dr.: The Northeast District

Memorial to Fallen Officers. The memorial consists of a small plaza displaying the police badges of the five officers from the Northeast District killed in the line of duty.

● Take Harford Rd. southwest back to your starting point at Lake Montebello.

POINTS OF INTEREST (START TO FINISH)

Lake Montebello Lake Dr.

Columbus Monument Harford Rd. and Walther Ave.

Northeast District Memorial to Fallen Officers Harford Rd. and Parkside Dr.

ROUTE SUMMARY

1. Start at Lake Montebello.
2. Walk the lake loop.
3. Cross Harford Rd. at the intersection of Harford Rd., Montebello Terr., and Chesterfield Ave.
4. Pick up Herring Run Trail through Herring Run Park.
5. Take a left on Belair Rd. and pick up Herring Run Trail on the north side of Herring Run.
6. Go under Harford Rd. and take a right on the service road.
7. Take the path from the parking area to a left onto Harford Rd.
8. Cross Harford Rd. past Walther Ave. to visit the Columbus and Fallen Officers Memorials.
9. Take Harford Rd. back to Lake Montebello.

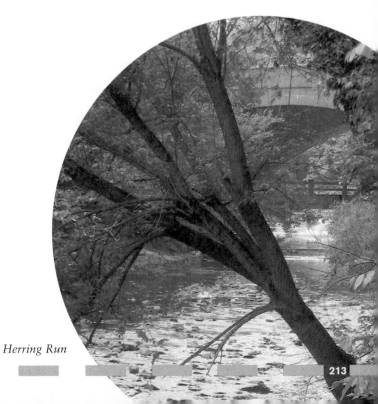

Herring Run

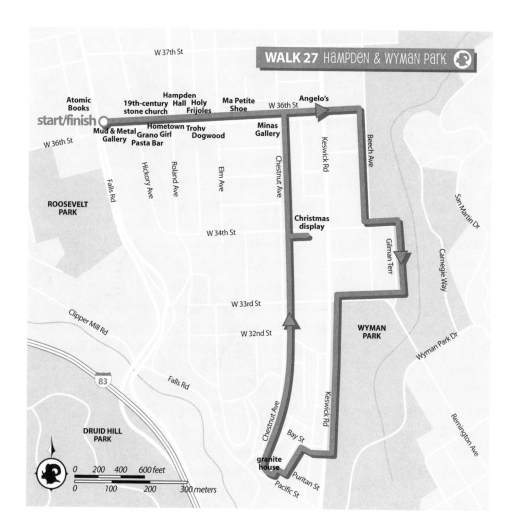

W 37th St

Atomic
Books

start/finish

Mud & Metal
Gallery

19th-century
stone church

Hampden
Hall Holy
Frijoles

Hometown
Grano Girl
Pasta Bar

Trohv
Dogwood

Ma Petite
Shoe

Angelo's

W 36th St

Minas
Gallery

W 36th St

Falls Rd

Hickory Ave

Roland Ave

Elm Ave

Chestnut Ave

Keswick Rd

Beech Ave

San Martin Dr

ROOSEVELT
PARK

W 34th St

Christmas
display

Gilman Terr

Carnegie Way

W 33rd St

W 32nd St

WYMAN
PARK

Wyman Park Dr

Clipper Mill Rd

Falls Rd

Chestnut Ave

Bay St

Keswick Rd

Remington Ave

DRUID HILL
PARK

83

granite
house

Puritan St

Pacific St

0   200   400   600 feet

0   100   200   300 meters

27 HAMPDEN & WYMAN PARK: HOME OF THE HONS

BOUNDARIES: **W. 36th St., Beech Ave., Gilman Terr., W. 33rd St., Chestnut Ave.**
DISTANCE: **2.3 miles**
DIFFICULTY: **Easy to moderate**
PARKING: **Street parking all along route**
PUBLIC TRANSIT: **Hampden Shuttle; MTA bus #27 runs along W. 36th St. and stops on Keswick Rd. as well as Chestnut Ave.**

Some locals will roll their eyes and mutter about the overplayed and commercialized Hon phenomenon. Others will lament that this once pure form of Baltimore hospitality has been so often parodied that it's lost its meaning. For those not in the know, Hon is the ubiquitous and indigenous Baltimore term of endearment. That traditional greeting, as in "Hey, Hon," has typified this corner of Baltimore for generations. It conjures up old ladies with beehive hair-dos and cat's-eye glasses, an easy mark for parody. However, let's not forget that it also signi-fies a sincere warmth. You're never a stranger in Hampden, not when you're called "hon." The annual Honfest, held on Hampden's main strip every June, and a public dispute over copyrights to the word itself, have thrust the term and all that goes with it into the spotlight. It has led many to mourn an earlier, simpler time, when Hampden was more like . . . well, Hampden. True, if you grew up here even 20 years ago and hadn't been back since, you would probably not recognize the place. But not all progress is bad. Though glorified as a center of Baltimore kitsch, Hampden has certainly had its recent problems. The disappear-ance of many blue-collar manufacturing jobs meant hard times for this neighborhood, but a renewal along 36th St. has brought not a wave of crass gentrification, but a status as one of Baltimore's most eclectic and interesting areas. Yes, the Hons are still here, but now, so it seems, is everyone else. On this walk, take in the new face of Hampden, plus some of the very old and a bit of neighboring Wyman Park as well.

● Begin on W. 36th St., at Falls Rd., in the heart of Hampden. Because of its proximity to the Jones Falls Valley and the many mills there (see Walk 28: Woodberry and Walk 22: Falls Road Turnpike), Hampden had been a center of mill work and manufacturing for more than 200 years. The first houses in what is now considered Hampden were erect-ed as early as 1802. The mills employed waves of newly arrived immigrants; over the decades, Hampden's population swelled with mostly Germans and Poles. You'll see that reflected even today in the family names of many Hampdenites. But the neighborhood was named for a Brit, one John Hampden, a member of Parliament who in 1637 led a protest against a levy, claiming it constituted taxation without representation.

● Before you head down Hampden's main commercial strip, check out Atomic Books, right behind you at 3620 Falls Rd. The store's slogan, "Literary Finds for Mutated Minds" tells you all you need to know. You might run into director John Waters here; he picks up his fan mail at Atomic Books. Waters has always been a big Hampden booster, and he celebrated the neighborhood in his 1998 film, *Pecker*, staring Edward Furlong and Christina Ricci. Virtually all of the locations for that movie are in this neighborhood. Hampden also gets some treatment in the critically acclaimed 2009 novel *American Rust*, by author Philipp Meyer, who grew up on W. 36th St.

● Head east down W. 36th St., known locally as The Avenue. This street has always been Hampden's main commercial drag. For 150 years, Hampden residents could and did shop for all their needs here; mill and manufacturing jobs were abundant and reliable. But as these dried up, so did the businesses along The Avenue. By the 1970s, the area had become a depressing no-go zone, full of boarded-up windows, public drunkenness, and petty crime. But Hampden and The Avenue were too good to stay down for long. By the early 1990s, businesses began moving back in. Today, it's a flourishing area, full of eclectic shops and restaurants. There are simply too many businesses to list here, so take your time traveling along The Avenue as you move from west to east toward Wyman Park. Here are some highlights (keep in mind this is not an exhaustive list—in addition to the below, you'll find a bunch of antiques stores, yoga studios, and even an organic hair salon; keep your eyes open for other places of interest and visit the Hampden Village Merchants' Association website at hampden merchants.com):

Mud & Metal Gallery (1121 W. 36th St.) Sculptures and ceramics for the home.

13.5% Wine Bar (1117 W. 36th St.) Getting accolades as one of Baltimore's best new bars.

The Golden West Café (1105 W. 36th St.) Long a local favorite. New Mexican food served with a decidedly bohemian air. (They'll kick you out if you're on your cell phone.)

On W. 36th St., just after Hickory St., is a 19th-century stone church, terribly damaged in a 1999 fire, but recently restored and awaiting new use.

Grano Pasta Bar (1031 W. 36th St.) This tiny place seats a maximum of 10 people. They offer a limited number of pastas and a limited number of sauces, and they do each one to something close to perfection. You choose the combo and watch them make it. (If you want an expanded menu and more sit-down options, but the same great quality and service, head a few blocks to Grano Emporio, at 3547 Chestnut Ave., just off W. 36th St.)

Café Hon (1002 W. 36th St.) You can't miss it. Just look for the enormous, two-story pink flamingo hanging above the entrance. Locally famous for the Hon trademark flap (see "Back Story" on next page) and for hosting celebrity chef Gordon Ramsay for an episode of *Kitchen Nightmares*.

Hampden Hall (corner of W. 36th St. and Roland Ave.) This 1882 building formerly served as a veterans' meeting hall. Check out the amazing mural facing W. 36th St. on the top floor. Dr. Bob Hieronimus, radio broadcaster and muralist, painted it. Hieronimus became famous in the late 1960s and early 1970s for his psychedelic murals and other work—his painted Volkswagen bus at Woodstock became an endearing symbol of that festival. Hieronimus painted this mural in 1975 for the upcoming bicentennial; in it, he honors Hampden's two Congressional Medal of Honor recipients from WWII. On the bottom right, you'll see the artist's homage to the Hampden Trolley Line of 1885, the nation's first trolley line, which used to run up and down these very streets.

Hampden mural

Back Story

Every year in late spring/early summer, The Avenue hosts the annual Honfest, a celebration of all things Hon. It began in 1994 as a paean to those working women of Baltimore who tossed around the term of endearment to anyone they came across. But its uniqueness and laugh-at-itself fun has made Honfest a national curiosity. It has been covered by everyone from the *New York Times* to Rachael Ray's *Tasty Travels*, from the *Nightly News with Brian Williams* to the *Los Angeles Times*, from HGTV to CNN. But a flap over the term darkened 2011's festival. The owner of the nearby Café Hon, it turns out, had trademarked the word. As one can imagine, the local protest was loud and vociferous. By the time dust had settled, the offending party had apologized (and reminded people of how her efforts have helped to transform Hampden into a tourist attraction—true enough). Now that feelings have been mended, everyone can go back to enjoying the four-block-long street party.

During the festival, women in outrageous leopard print, spandex, and bright blue eye shadow, and with gravity-defying beehive hairdos compete for the honorific Miss Hon. The festival also celebrates the local dialect, Bawlmorese, Baltimore's unique traditional accent. Bawlmorese even got its turn on the *Voice of America* in 2011 with the program, "Hey, Hon, Ready to Learn How They Talk in Baltimore?"

Hometown Girl (1001 W. 36th St.) All kinds of Baltimore-centric souvenirs. And a real soda fountain too.

Trohv (921 W. 36th St.) Wonderful furniture and home accessories store with some amazing pieces. (Locals might know this place by its original name, Red Tree.)

Dogwood (911 W. 36th St.) A restaurant with a mission, employing people "who are transitioning from addiction, incarceration, homelessness, and/or underemployment." Come for the food; it's simply terrific, evidenced by its consistent garnering of Best of Baltimore awards.

Holy Frijoles (908 W. 36th St.) Cheap but good Mexican eats. Long a local favorite.

Ma Petite Shoe (832 W. 36th St.) It advertises "Shoes and Chocolate"—what more could a woman want?

Minas Gallery (815 W. 36th St.) Art gallery that hosts a monthly literary reading series frequented by some of Baltimore's best writers.

- Continue on W. 36th St. until it ends at Beech Ave. (If you haven't already eaten and pizza is your thing, check out Angelo's, at the corner of W. 36th St. and Keswick Rd., one block before Beech Ave. Angelo's claims to serve the largest slice in the world; while that can't be proven, it's most certainly the largest in the city.) When you hit Beech Ave., you'll see a terrific green space in front of you. This is Wyman Park. Take advantage and head into the park; you'll inevitably find some game or another in full swing—most probably that Baltimore institution, lacrosse. You can also head straight, where you'll eventually hit a stream, Stoney Run. In the 18th and 19th centuries, two flour mills operated nearby along the stream. Up the hill on the other side of Stoney Run is the campus of Johns Hopkins University.

- When you've renewed yourself in the park, go back to Beech Ave. and follow it south, paralleling Wyman Park to your left. Narrow two-story houses line the street facing the park. The neighborhood of Wyman Park is generally understood to be a rather narrow strip east of Keswick Rd. to the park and between 33rd St. and 40th St. The park itself remains the neighborhood's focal point. Though industry and attendant taverns and other services have been in this area since the 18th century, and you'll find some houses from the late 1880s, the majority of Wyman Park's residences weren't built until the early to mid-20th century.

- At W. 34th St., take a left and then a quick right as W. 34th swings around to become Gilman Terr., with its collection of handsome brick porch-front homes. Gilman Terr. soon ends at the confluence of Remington Ave. and W. 33rd. St. Go west on W. 33rd St. and take the first left onto Keswick Rd.

- Follow Keswick Rd. past Singer Ave. to the next right, Bay St. Once on Bay St., you'll notice immediately that things look very different from where you've come. That is because you have entered the Stone Hill section of Hampden. This National Historic District is the remarkably intact complex of mill workers' houses, all built of rugged and beautiful granite between 1845 and 1847 for workers of the Mount Vernon Mills (see Walk 22: Falls Road Turnpike). Take an immediate left on Worth St. to stay in this extraordinary enclave.

- Stay on Worth St. by crossing Puritan St. Worth St. becomes Pacific St. at an amazing granite house to your right. This house, 732 Pacific St., was the summer home of the Quaker abolitionist Elisha Tyson, owner of the Mount Vernon Mills and organizer of safe houses for runaway slaves. His philanthropy knew no bounds; he founded the Baltimore House of Industry in 1804, providing job training to the poor; the Baltimore Society to Protect Free Negroes in 1810; and the Baltimore House of Refuge in 1817. When Tyson died in 1824, it is said that as many as 10,000 free blacks joined the procession. The house's construction dates to sometime between 1790 and 1804; it eventually became the mill superintendent's home. The house was painstakingly preserved between 2005 and 2009. The restoration project has garnered much attention in local and regional preservationist circles, but remember that this is a private property and respect it accordingly.

- Follow Pacific St. until you come to a stop sign, where the road merges into Chestnut Ave. Take Chestnut Ave. right. You will no doubt notice old mill buildings to your left, overlooking the Jones Falls Valley. Follow Chestnut Ave. four blocks to W. 34th St. To your right is the 700 block of W. 34th St.

- If it's December and it's evening, you're in for an enormous treat. If it isn't, make sure to come back at that time. While this row of houses might look unassuming at any other time of year, during Christmas the residents of this block turn their little stretch into a self-anointed Miracle on 34th Street. The display of lights and decorations defies description; it simply has to be seen to be believed. Featured in regional, national, and even international media, this Miracle on 34th Street has seen visitors from all over the world who come to gawk at the extraordinary display. Thousands and thousands of lights, inflatable creatures, moving trains, music, angels, and more create enough kinetic energy to light a city block; the effect it has on visitors is something to behold. Even for those of us who come check it out every year, it's great fun to simply watch visitors walk through, gawking and smiling and taking family pictures and shepherding amazed children. It truly is a reminder of what the season is all about, and the residents who live here surely deserve thanks for their gift.

● Return to Chestnut Ave. and head north. The architecture in this part of Hampden is mostly Federal and Greek Revival. While the brick houses here were built primarily for mill workers, you'll pass some larger stone homes; these were built for mill managers, upper-level staff, and their families. In four blocks, you will come to W. 36th St. Take a left to return toward Falls Rd., where you began.

POINTS OF INTEREST (START TO FINISH)

Atomic Books atomicbooks.com, 3620 Falls Rd., 410-662-4444

Angelo's 3600 Keswick Rd., 410-235-2595

Stone Hill Historic District Pacific, Puritan, Bay, Field, and Worth Sts.

Miracle on 34th Street 700 Block of W. 34th St.

For more information, visit honfest.net and hampdenmerchants.com

ROUTE SUMMARY

1. Start at Falls Rd. and W. 36th St.; walk east on W. 36th St.
2. Turn right onto Beech Ave.
3. Turn left onto W. 34th St.
4. Turn right onto Gilman Terr.
5. Turn right onto W. 33rd. St.
6. Turn left onto Keswick Rd.
7. Turn right onto Bay St.
8. Turn left onto Worth St.
9. Stay on Worth St. as it becomes Pacific St.
10. Merge right onto Chestnut Ave.
11. Turn right onto the 700 block of W. 34th St. (if Christmastime).
12. Return to W. 36th St. via Chestnut Ave.

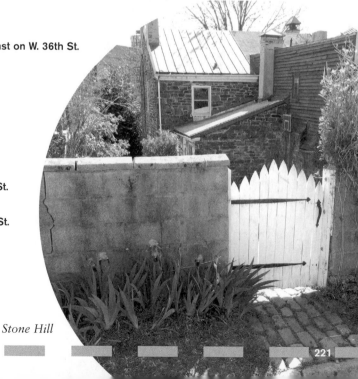

Stone Hill

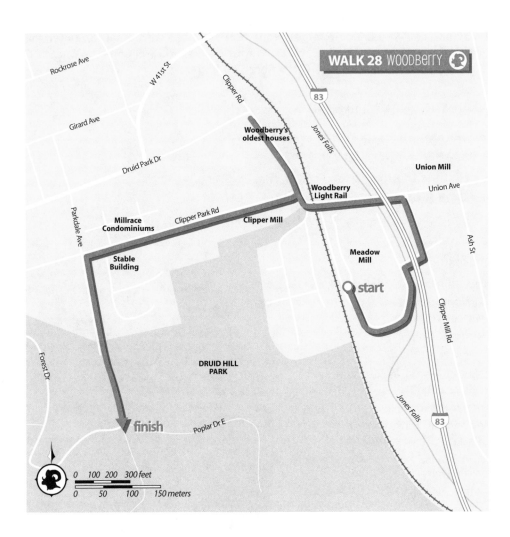

Rockrose Ave

W 41st St

Clipper Rd

83

Girard Ave

Jones Falls

Woodberry's
oldest houses

Druid Park Dr

Union Mill

Union Ave

Woodberry
Light Rail

Parkdale Ave

Millrace
Condominiums

Clipper Park Rd

Clipper Mill

Meadow
Mill

Stable
Building

Ash St

start

Clipper Mill Rd

DRUID HILL
PARK

Forest Dr

Jones Falls

83

finish

Poplar Dr E

0   100 200   300 feet

0   50   100   150 meters

28 WOODBErry: UrBan revitalization Done right

BOUNDARIES: **Union Ave., Clipper Rd., Clipper Mill Rd., Parkdale Ave.**
DISTANCE: **1.25 miles**
DIFFICULTY: **Easy**
PARKING: **At Meadow Mill or along Union Ave.**
PUBLIC TRANSIT: **Woodberry Light Rail, MTA bus #22 stops at Druid Park Dr. and 41st St. and Druid Park Dr. and Parkdale Ave. MTA bus #98 (the Hampden Shuttle) stops at Druid Park Dr. and Clipper Rd.**

Woodberry remains one of Baltimore's unique neighborhoods. When mill production contributed significantly to Baltimore's economy in the mid-19th to early 20th century, Woodberry was an epicenter. Because of its strategic location along rail lines and the Jones Falls, good solid jobs were plentiful, and hundreds of families set up here. But the coming decline in manufacturing brought hard times for Woodberry. The mills shuttered one by one and fell into disrepair. But good times are here once again; the rebirth of these extraordinary structures means Woodberry sits on the cusp of being Baltimore's next great place (if it isn't already). The neighborhood is known today for its encompassing grand historic mills, Television Hill, and the presence of the stone houses built in the 19th century to house workers for the nearby mills. This walk takes in three of those mills—Meadow Mill, Union Mill, and the fabulous Clipper Mill. The latter is one of the greatest examples of urban renewal of its kind in the United States. Throw in the Jones Falls and a bit of Druid Hill Park, and this walk takes in some of Baltimore's iconic places.

● Begin at Meadow Mill, built in the 1870s by William Hooper and Sons. The Hooper name retained some prominence for years to come (note Hooper Ave. off Druid Park Dr. just one block north of Clipper Mill); onetime mill owner Alcaeus Hooper was elected mayor of Baltimore in 1895. Today, Meadow Mill hosts a popular athletic club, the terrific Stone Mill Bakery, the theater troupe Mobtown Players (mobtownplayers. com), and the Potters Guild of Baltimore (pottersguildofbaltimore.com). The latter captured the attention of Oscar-winning actress Melissa Leo, who used to stop by when she was a cast member on *Homicide: Life on the Street.*

● Cross the Jones Falls from the Meadow Mill parking lot and head left. But don't go so quickly; you're bound to see some interesting wildlife in the river. I've spotted many herons, fish, and turtles, and once almost stepped on a large, poisonous northern copperhead sunning itself on the banks.

● As you reach Union Ave., you'll see Union Mill, Maryland's largest stone mill. Erected in 1866, the mill was at one time the largest producer of cotton duck (canvas) in the world. This duck was turned into sailcloth that powered the iconic Baltimore clippers of the 1800s. Like the other nearby mills, Union had closed down by the mid-20th century and fell into neglect. Today, it has been reborn as an urban oasis, meeting green standards and offering more than 25,000 square feet of office space to non-profits, as well as discounted residences for Baltimore city teachers.

● Turn left on Union Ave. and approach the Woodberry Light Rail stop. Cross the tracks and head right on Clipper Rd. As you walk up the hill, you'll see Woodberry's oldest houses—stone beauties from the mid-19th century, built for mill workers. Woodberry proper stretches all the way up to Television Hill, where you'll see the towers that transmit broadcasts for five Baltimore television stations.

● Turn around and head back toward the Light Rail. On your right will be the entrance to Clipper Mill, along Clipper Park Rd. The entrance is marked by a memorial to Eric Dorian Schaefer, a city firefighter who tragically lost his life on September 16, 1995, battling a massive blaze that swept through a large section of the Clipper Mill complex. As you will see as you walk, the complex has many original buildings, but new construction marks the places where the fire destroyed some 19th-century structures.

Clipper Mill has been an impressive place ever since its inception along the banks of the Jones Falls 150 years ago. According to the history section on clippermill baltimore.com, among the notable aspects of Clipper Mill's past include: it once contained the country's largest machine manufacturing plant and the world's largest lathe, "capable of turning out a wheel [of cotton canvas] sixty feet in diameter." Additionally, the plant cast the bronze pillars that support the U.S. Capitol dome. Now, the site houses an eclectic collection of offices, shops, galleries, and studios, including those for glassblowers, jewelers, sculptors, and architectural metalworkers.

It also includes one of Baltimore's hottest restaurants (and deservedly so), the farm-to-table Woodberry Kitchen. Green-conscious residences also populate the area.

- As you walk through the Clipper Mill complex from the firefighters' memorial, you will be looking at the large stone structure on the right that is the original Poole & Hunt building. Dating from 1856, it is the oldest surviving building in the complex. The brick-and-stone section with the cupola closest to Clipper Road was a 1905 addition and housed the millwright's office.

- Directly across the street, to the left of where you are standing, are the Millrace Condominiums. While small sections of the 1853 Machine Shop still stand, the original building burned down in 1995 (see firefighters' memorial, above).

- Continuing on, the massive stone building to the right is the original Foundry (1870), which now houses studios, Woodberry Kitchen, and other offic-   es.

- The 1890 Assembly building sits across the street and is home to offices and residences (with a pretty cool Roman bath–style swimming pool in between). The Assembly building was also badly damaged in the 1995 fire. But the soaring ceilings (80 feet high) still remain, giving a good sense of the scale of the place.

- Next to the Assembly building is the Tractor building (1916), awaiting renovation into more residential and office space. Despite its neglected appearance (especially in contrast to the renovated Assembly build-ing next door), the Tractor building does not detract in the slightest from the complex. In fact, the mix of new and old, refurbished and deteriorating,

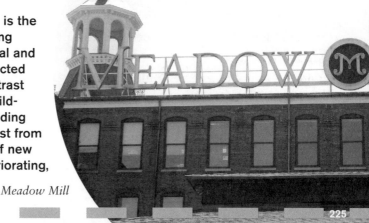

Meadow Mill

is fascinating to observe. Here is a grand opportunity to see what once was, what is now, and what is coming.

● Continuing on, the small stone building on the left is the original Stable building (1890), where the wagons and horses used for transport were housed. Behind the Stable building, down Woodberry Ave., sits Overlook Clipper Mill, a cluster of new residential green constructions.

● After you've poked around Clipper Mill, continue east on Clipper Park Rd. to a left on Parkdale Ave. (the next left after Woodberry). This short road dead-ends at the Jones Falls Trail (JFT) in Druid Hill Park. Druid Hill Park is a wonderful urban playground, home to the Maryland Zoo, the Rawlings Conservatory and Botanic Gardens, and a ton of recreational-activity sites. The JFT in this section travels a series of short switchbacks and heads deep into the park toward the Druid Hill disc golf course. Obviously, how far you wish to travel on the JFT is up to you, but note that a separate walk in this book (Walk 23: Druid Hill Park) takes in this section of the JFT plus the rest of the park. No matter how far you go, when you are done at the park, retrace your steps to Parkdale.

● Turn right on Clipper Park Rd. and head back to Meadow Mill.

POINTS OF INTEREST (START TO FINISH)

Meadow Mill Clipper Mill Rd.

Union Mill theunionmill.com, 1500 Union Ave., 443-682-9945

Clipper Mill clippermillbaltimore.com

Woodberry Kitchen woodberrykitchen.com, 2010 Clipper Park Rd., 410-464-8000

Druid Hill Park/Jones Falls Trail (Friends of Druid Hill Park) druidhillpark.org, 443-469-8274

route summary

1. Begin at Meadow Mill.
2. Cross the Jones Falls and take a left toward Union Mill.
3. Turn left on Union Ave.
4. Turn right on Clipper Rd. and follow it to the stone houses.
5. Turn around on Clipper Rd. and go right on Clipper Park Rd.
6. Turn left on Parkdale Ave.
7. Reverse all directions to return to Meadow Mill.

Connecting the Walks

At the end of this walk, when you reach Druid Hill Park from Parkdale Ave., you can easily continue to take in the walk at Druid Hill Park (Walk 23). You will be entering the park at a different location from the Druid Hill Park walk description, but it's easy enough to stitch them together without losing your way.

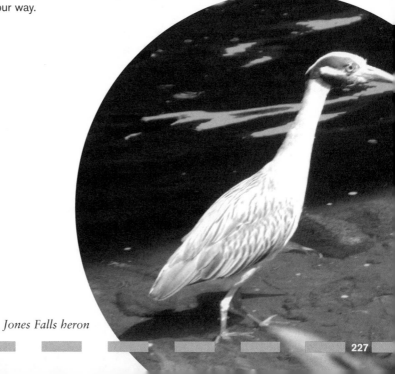

Jones Falls heron

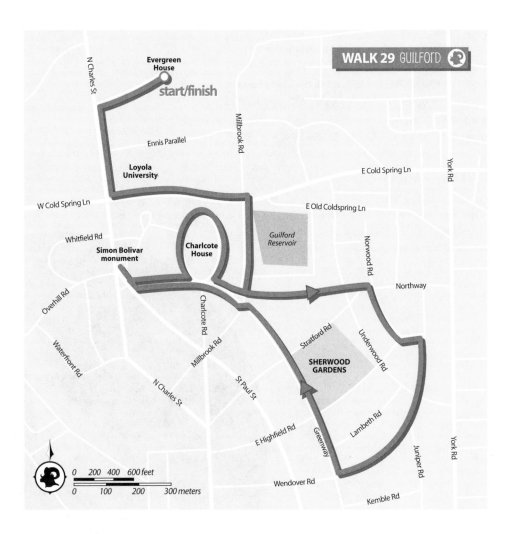

Evergreen
House

start/finish

N Charles St

Millbrook Rd

Ennis Parallel

**Loyola
University**

E Cold Spring Ln

York Rd

W Cold Spring Ln

E Old Coldspring Ln

Whitfield Rd

*Guilford
Reservoir*

Norwood Rd

**Simon Bolivar
monument**

**Charlcote
House**

Northway

Overhill Rd

Charlcote Rd

Stratford Rd

Underwood Rd

Waterfront Rd

Millbrook Rd

**SHERWOOD
GARDENS**

N Charles St

St Paul St

Lambeth Rd

Juniper Rd

York Rd

E Highfield Rd

Greenway

Wendover Rd

Kemble Rd

0   200   400   600 feet

0   100   200   300 meters

29 GUILFORD: YeaH, IT'S PreTTY NICe

BOUNDARIES: N. Charles St., Cold Spring Ln., Wendover Rd., Greenway, Charlcote Pl.
DISTANCE: 3 miles
DIFFICULTY: Moderate
PARKING: At Evergreen House (or to stay entirely in the residential section of Guilford, along Millbrook Rd. adjacent to the Guilford Reservoir)
PUBLIC TRANSIT: MTA bus #11 runs along N. Charles St. Use the Loyola College stop and head north, passing Cold Spring Ln. There are also stops at St. Paul St./N. Charles St., St. Paul St. and Greenway, and St. Paul St. and Charlcote Pl. MTA bus #33 stops at Cold Spring Ln. and Millbrook Rd.

Many civic boosters claim their own neighborhoods as Baltimore's prettiest. With so many varied neighborhoods in the city, what constitutes the most attractive is difficult to quantify. But one thing seems undisputed: Guilford, if not Baltimore's prettiest neighborhood, is certainly one of its toniest. And it has been for 100 years now, earning itself a designation on the National Register of Historic Places. Walking through this enclave is a delightful experience because what you see isn't vanity and ostentation—it's quality. The homes are of solid and thoughtful construction, with no shortcuts taken in creating magnificent edifices of stone, brick, and stucco. Some of Baltimore's most prominent 19th- and early 20th-century architects designed many of these Guilford homes: Laurence Hall Fowler, W. D. Lamdin, Edward L. Palmer, John Russell Pope, and Bayard Turnbull among them. The architecture reflects mostly European revival styles, such as Italianate, Tudor, and Renaissance. Throw in the gorgeous and public Sherwood Gardens, with its 80,000 tulip bulbs, and Guilford gets my vote for prettiest.

● Begin at the Evergreen House, part of the Johns Hopkins University's museum system and on the National Register of Historic Places. The mansion was built in the late 19th century by the Garrett family, made fabulously wealthy in railroading. The mansion itself is an absolute beauty with almost 50 rooms and more than 50,000 pieces from the Garretts' amazing possessions remaining in view. The 26 manicured acres and gardens don't disappoint, either.

● After Evergreen, walk down the driveway to Charles St. and turn left, taking the first left onto Cold Spring Ln. You'll be paralleling Loyola University. The university, recently renamed after a century and a half of being known as Loyola College, is part of the national consortium of Jesuit colleges and universities. Begun in 1852, it is one of the oldest of that group. Poke around the campus a bit, as some of the original Gothic buildings are quite lovely.

● Continue on Cold Spring Ln. to the first right onto Millbrook Rd. The hill to the left hides the Guilford Reservoir.

● You'll soon reach the confluence of Millbrook Rd, Northway, and Greenway. You've now entered the residential area of Guilford, and its beauty is immediately evident. Tasteful houses of solid and varied construction, wide tree-lined streets, and a definite air of exclusivity dominate. This is no happy accident; Guilford at one time came under the planning auspices of the Roland Park Company, and the same landscape design principles put into place in that beautiful neighborhood apply here as well (see Walk 30: Roland Park). The streets follow natural contours, and mature trees, green spaces, and parks are abundant.

● You will enjoy simply wandering around the streets of Guilford, but to follow this walk, which roughly takes in the neighborhood's farthest reaches, take a left on Northway.

● Continue on Northway to a right on Norwood Rd, passing Underwood Rd. No doubt you'll notice an extraordinary green space to your right as you walk; this is the locally famous Sherwood Gardens—more on that later.

● Norwood Rd. ends at Marlow Rd., where you will take a left.

● Then take a right on Wendover Rd. You'll soon pass Underwood Rd. again. If you are interested in seeing where the inimitable author Ogden Nash lived, take a right on Underwood to his old house at #4205. Return to Wendover Rd. and when you reach Greenway, take another right, heading north. Pass Lambeth Rd. and Highfield Rd., and you'll soon reach the 4100 block of Greenway. The property at 4100 Greenway is the site of the original Guilford Mansion, razed in 1914. A certain William McDonald built the old mansion in the middle of the 19th century. (History relates that McDonald served time in Fort McHenry for using the tower of his mansion to signal messages to Confederate troops during the Civil War.) The property eventually passed into the hands of Arunah Abell, founder of the *Baltimore Sun*. Also on this block, bordered by Stratford Rd. to the north, is Sherwood Gardens.

Take time to linger here, at Sherwood Gardens, which is justifiably famous for its springtime profusion of tulips. Some 80,000 bulbs are planted annually, and around the end of April into the beginning of May the show is nothing short of spectacular. But it's lovely any time of year. Offering more than 6 acres with plenty of shade and benches, Sherwood Gardens makes a great place to spend an hour or two.

- Fully rejuvenated after a pause at Sherwood Gardens, you should continue heading north on Greenway until it ends at St. Paul St. This is a busy thoroughfare and it breaks the solitude a bit. Immediately to the right is one of Baltimore's many monuments; this time it's Simon Bolivar, the Great Liberator of much of South America. He is honored with a bust on Bedford Square.

- Return to Greenway and take it to the circle on Charlcote Pl. In the middle of the circle sits the enormous Charlcote House, designed and built in 1914 by John Russell Pope, who also designed the Jefferson Memorial and the West Wing of the National Gallery of Art in Washington, D.C.

- Continue on the circle around Charlcote Pl. until it ends at Greenway and take a left. You'll very soon come to Millbrook Rd., where you can retrace your steps to the Evergreen House.

POINTS OF INTEREST (START TO FINISH)

Evergreen Museum & Library museums.jhu.edu/evergreen.php, 4545 N. Charles St., 410-516-0341

Loyola University of Maryland loyola.edu, 4501 N. Charles St., 410-617-2000 or 800-221-9107

Sherwood Gardens guilfordassociation.org/sherwood, bracketed by Greenway, Stratford Rd., Highfield Rd., and Underwood Rd.

route summary

1. Start at the Evergreen House.
2. Turn left onto Charles St.
3. Turn left onto Cold Spring Ln.
4. Turn right onto Millbrook Rd.
5. Turn left onto Northway.
6. Turn right on Norwood Rd.
7. Turn left on Marlow Rd.
8. Turn right on Wendover Rd.
9. Turn right on Greenway.
10. Turn right on St. Paul St./Bedford Pl.
11. Return to Greenway.
12. Turn left on Charlcote Pl.
13. Turn left on Greenway.
14. Turn left on Millbrook Rd.
15. Turn left on Cold Spring Ln.
16. Turn right on Charles St.
17. Turn right to Evergreen House.

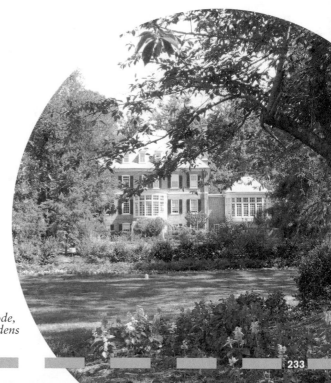

Typical Guilford abode,
seen through Sherwood Gardens

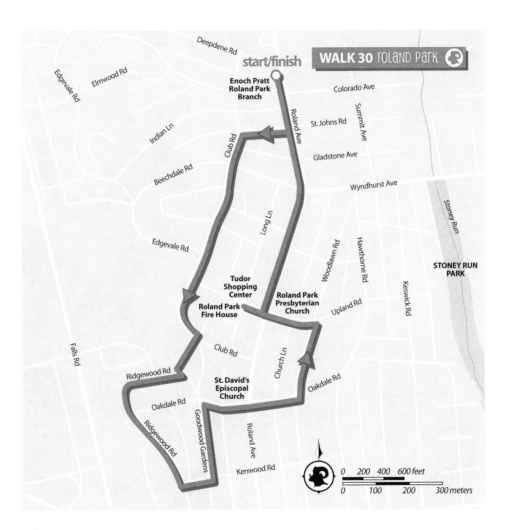

start/finish

WALK 30 roLaND Park

Deepdene Rd

Enoch Pratt
Roland Park
Branch

Colorado Ave

Edgevale Rd

Elmwood Rd

St. Johns Rd

Summit Ave

Roland Ave

Indian Ln

Club Rd

Gladstone Ave

Beechdale Rd

Wyndhurst Ave

Stoney Run

Edgevale Rd

Long Ln

STONEY RUN
PARK

Woodlawn Rd

Hawthorne Rd

Keswick Rd

Tudor
Shopping
Center

Roland Park
Presbyterian
Church

Roland Park
Fire House

Upland Rd

Falls Rd

Club Rd

Church Ln

Ridgewood Rd

St. David's
Episcopal
Church

Oakdale Rd

Oakdale Rd

Goodwood Gardens

Roland Ave

Ridgewood Rd

Kenwood Rd

0   200   400   600 feet

0   100   200   300 meters

30 roLanD ParK: CITY BeauTIFuL

BOUNDARIES: **Blackberry Ln., Club Rd., Ridgewood Rd., Kenwood Rd., Woodlawn Rd.**
DISTANCE: **2.4 miles**
DIFFICULTY: **Moderate**
PARKING: **Street parking all along route**
PUBLIC TRANSIT: **MTA buses #s 27, 44, and 61 stop along Roland Ave.**

Roland Park is in some respects the perfect "suburban" neighborhood. Of course, after Roland Park's annexation to Baltimore City in 1918, it isn't really a suburban neighborhood at all, but rather one of those glorious North Baltimore urban neighborhoods that clings tenaciously to its country feel. Originally conceived as a streetcar suburb linked to downtown by the rail line, it today retains that far-flung, world-apart feel, an oasis of beauty with winding, tree-lined streets and secret pathways that just scream for ambling, moseying, exploring. The Roland Park Company developed Roland Park between 1890 and 1920 from the acquisition of two large bordering estates. The original plans laid out two plats, the first designed by George Kessler, a famed architect associated with the City Beautiful movement. City Beautiful emphasized physical beauty—flowers, streams, rolling hills, structures that worked with the landscape instead of against it—as a means of creating better and more civil societies. The famed landscape architect Frederick Law Olmsted Jr. designed Plat 2 and carried the City Beautiful mantle. As the 20th century arrived, Roland Park expanded to include four more plats, laying out the neighborhood boundaries as they are today. The 1893 Lake Roland Elevated Railway allowed residents to make a direct trip to City Hall downtown. The addition of the country's first strip mall made Roland Park a self-sustaining enclave where upper-middle-class Baltimoreans could enjoy the best of their neighborhood. From the beginning, residents were required to pay levies designed for no other purpose than the continued maintenance and ongoing beautification of the neighborhood. They're called Homeowners' Associations today, of course, but in the late 19th century, it was a novel idea. What's wonderful about Roland Park today is that it hasn't lost one iota of its charm. Indeed, it is little surprise that well over a hundred years since the neighborhood's inception, Roland Park is quite literally a case study in urban-planning textbooks and classrooms all over the world.

● **Roland Park is rather large, stretching to Northern Pkwy. in the north, all the way to the edge of Johns Hopkins University in the south, Stoney Run to the east, and**

Falls Rd. to the west. There is little of it that isn't beautiful, and as with several other neighborhood-centered walks in this book (Homeland, Guilford, etc.), you are definitely encouraged to veer off the suggested route here and discover the side streets and connector paths that help to make Roland Park one of the most beautiful planned neighborhoods anywhere.

This walk is concentrated in the heart of Roland Park. It's logical then to begin at one of the neighborhood's central meeting points, the Roland Park branch of the Enoch Pratt Free Library. The original library was built in 1924, but the structure was renovated and expanded in 2008; the library now boasts some 9,500 square feet and possesses some stunning etched-glass panes by local artist Dan Herman. There was some controversy surrounding this expansion, however, in that it came at a time when the city was closing other branches. However, if customer usage is any argument for expansion, Roland Park deserved it. The library's usage numbers are astronomical, a sign of this affluent neighborhood's residents being not only well heeled but generally very well educated, curious, and immensely appreciative of their local library. Roland Park does therefore make a logical home for some of the city's finest private schools; Gilman, Roland Park Country, Friends, Calvert, and Bryn Mawr all call Roland Park home, while Boys' Latin is just outside of Roland Park's boundaries. Additionally, Roland Park Elementary and Middle have long been considered among the better public schools in the city.

● From the library, head south on Roland Ave., passing Longwood Rd. and Indian Ln., and take a right onto St. John's Rd. The impressively varied and always beautiful architecture pops out immediately; this is a late-Victorian neighborhood, with late-19th- and early 20th-century revival styles: Greek, Tudor, Italianate, Queen Anne, Shingle, Gothic, Georgian, and Regency. But you'll also find Arts and Crafts, bungalows, and a host of Spanish and Mediterranean Revival houses as well. What is also immediately evident is the fruition of the original architects' vision; the houses and streets here work with the natural landscape, moving in twists and turns and never impeding the earth's natural flow.

● Take a left onto Club Rd. You will be following this road for the next seven blocks, so take time to really enjoy the surroundings (and, if the mood strikes, take time also to explore some side streets). When you reach Upland Rd., you'll see the Baltimore

Country Club to your right. The club was founded here in 1898 and gained some national recognition the following year when it hosted the U.S. Open, then only in its fifth year. Follow the brick wall around the club and look for the little sign pointing you to Sunset Path. Take it right, down the hill, to see an extraordinary property. First, a note about this path. The Olmsteds constructed it, along with 17 others, to expedite foot traffic throughout the neighborhood in places where rolling hills made development of roads difficult. Instead of flattening the land or blasting through hillsides, the architects gave residents a series of almost magical passageways that kept the charm in and artificial obtrusiveness out. Sunset is named for the incredible views it affords of the sunset over Cylburn Arboretum, a mile or so in the distance. But Sunset is just one nicely named path (many carry the whiff of the English, which is not merely coincidental). The others: Climbing, Tintern, Shipton, St. Margaret's (bisected by a lovely little stream), Laurel, Squirrel, Litchfield, Hilltop, Brier, Tulip, Upland, Ten Oaks, Vanbiber, Kittery, Rye, Hepburn, and Audley End. Roland Park's Roads and Maintenance committee oversees the paths' maintenance, and they do a terrific job.

Decked with attractive signage, the paths zip through vegetation that is allowed to grow (to overgrow, in fact), but never encroach. The paths themselves are only wide enough for foot traffic, and it's common to see kids taking them on the way to school, or residents using them to get to the grocery. In winter, people even sled on them. To see a map of Roland Park path locations, visit rolandpark.org/civicleague/ documents/RPFootpaths.pdf

- The incredible stone house just off Sunset Path is called Rusty Rocks. (It's a private home, so don't snoop.) This was Roland Park Company President Edward H. Bouton's home. It was built in 1907 on the site of a quarry that supplied rocks for many of

Rusty Rocks

237

Back Story

Roland Park has quite a literary pedigree. The neighborhood serves as the setting for much of Anne Tyler's fiction and was used as the filming location of the movie adaptation of *The Accidental Tourist*. The poet Adrienne Rich grew up in Roland Park and attended the Roland Park Country School. She won the National Book Award for her 1974 book, *Diving into the Wreck*. In addition to her award-winning poetry, Rich was also well known for her activism, twice turning down invitations to the White House (from Bill Clinton and George W. Bush) for political reasons. Roland Park resident Alice Steinbach, who won many awards for her journalism, was a longtime writer for the *Baltimore Sun* and had her work distributed nationally through the *L.A. Times–Washington Post* wire service. Steinbach won a Pulitzer Prize for Feature Writing in 1985. Rich and Steinbach died within weeks of each other in early 2012. John Dos Passos (see Walk 32: Mount Washington) lived here for a while, and Ogden Nash lived just across Falls Rd. in Cross Keys, as well as in the sister neighborhood of Homeland. Walter Lord, who wrote *A Night to Remember*, a widely read account of the sinking of the *Titanic*, attended Gilman and grew up in the house at 4314 Roland Ave. Many other well-known and contemporary writers, such as Christopher Corbett *(The Poker Bride, Orphans Preferred)* and Jessica Anya Blau (*The Summer of Naked Swim Parties, Drinking Closer to Home*), make their homes today in Roland Park.

the houses in Roland Park. The Olmsted brothers designed the house, but Bouton considered the site unsuitable for sale. Today, the remaining rocks have been put to great use in constructing many terraces and walls.

● Continue to the end of the path where it meets Boulder Ln. and take a left. The intersection straight ahead is Boulder, Goodwood Gardens, and Ridgewood Rd. Take Ridgewood down the hill to the right. Ridgewood Rd. is one of Roland Park's absolute gems; the houses here, all varying in architecture and style, are simply beauties. Enormous, yes, but nothing ostentatious. Just solidly constructed, well-kept stunners.

And, as is the case elsewhere in this terrific neighborhood, the streets follow the natural contours of the land, and mature and leafy trees abound.

- When you reach Kenwood Rd, take a left. In another few hundred feet is Goodwood Gardens. Take a left onto this street and prepare to be wowed. Like Ridgewood, here you will find a collection of architectural masterpieces. Follow Goodwood Gardens to the next intersection, where you should take a right onto Oakdale Rd., passing the hundred-year-old and beautiful St. David's Episcopal Church on the corner. Once across Roland Ave., you'll pass an attractive stone church, now home to the North Baltimore Mennonite congregation.

- Take a left onto Woodlawn Rd. and follow it to the next intersection, which is Upland Rd. Take a left onto Upland. (Again, if the mood strikes, feel free to deviate from this route—which provides only a relatively small taste of Roland Park—and explore wherever your impulses lead you. For instance, heading right instead of left onto Upland will eventually take you to Stoney Run Park, with its namesake waterway, a lovely little ribbon of a stream winding through thick woods.)

- Approach Roland Ave. using Upland Rd. The church on your immediate right is the Roland Park Presbyterian Church, constructed in 1902. Fans of the actor Kevin Bacon will regard this church as a shrine; in his first film, Barry Levinson's *Diner* (1982), an inebriated Bacon sacks out in a manger and winds up punching some of the manger's residents; that scene was shot in front of this church.

- Cross Roland Ave. to check out the striking Tudor shopping center that is widely considered the country's first strip mall. This makes sense considering Roland Park's designation as the country's first planned neighborhood. This shopping center also has to be the country's most attractive strip mall. It was built in 1896, primarily because distance to downtown shopping made Roland Park seem particularly far-flung. With the shopping center, locals could stay in the neighborhood and get most of their errands done. The strip of Roland Ave. where the shopping center is located has always been designated as Roland Park's business district. This design separated it from other nearby planned communities, such as Guilford and Homeland, which are similar architecturally and in landscape-usage philosophy but lack a central business strip. The Roland Park Company's first office was in this building. Streetcars passed by this business center and then circled it to head back and forth from downtown. Today, the building, on the National Register of Historic Places, houses one of the more popular local restaurants, the French bistro Petit Louis.

● Continuing along Upland Rd., you'll pass the still-functioning Roland Park Fire House. It has been in continuous use since its construction in 1896, making it the city's oldest such firehouse. The apartment complex next to it at 4 Upland Rd. is where the Roland Park streetcar terminated. Various streetcars labored on until 1947, when buses and automobiles made this mode of transport a relic. Next up is the Roland Park Condominiums, housed in a beautiful building. The condos' garage once served as a community stable.

● Return to Roland Ave. by turning around and then heading left on Roland. The library, this walk's starting point, is seven blocks away. Roland Ave., despite being the main drag, is still rather nice, with beautiful homes lining both sides. But if you find that it's too busy for you, you can always take a parallel street on your way back to the library.

POINTS OF INTEREST (START TO FINISH)

Enoch Pratt Free Library, Roland Park Branch prattlibrary.org/locations/rolandpark, 5108 Roland Ave.

St. David's Episcopal Church stdavid.ang-md.org, 4700 Roland Ave., 410-467-0476

Roland Park Presbyterian Church rolandparkchurch.org, 4801 Roland Ave., 410-889-2000

Tudor Shopping Center Upland Rd. and Roland Ave.

Petit Louis petitlouis.com, 4800 Roland Ave., 410-366-9393

Roland Park Fire House Upland Rd.

ROUTE SUMMARY

1. Start at the Enoch Pratt Free Library, Roland Park branch, at 5108 Roland Ave.
2. Turn right onto St. John's Rd.
3. Turn left onto Club Rd.
4. Turn right onto Sunset Path.

5. Turn left onto Boulder Rd.
6. Turn right onto Ridgewood Rd.
7. Turn left onto Kenwood Rd.
8. Turn left onto Goodwood Gardens.
9. Turn right onto Oakdale Rd.
10. Turn left onto Woodlawn Rd.
11. Turn left onto Upland Rd.
12. Visit shopping center, fire house, and Roland Park Condominiums on Upland Rd.
13. Return to Roland Ave. and go left.
14. Follow Roland Ave. back to the library.

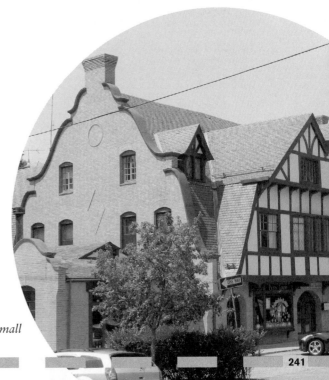

The country's first shopping mall

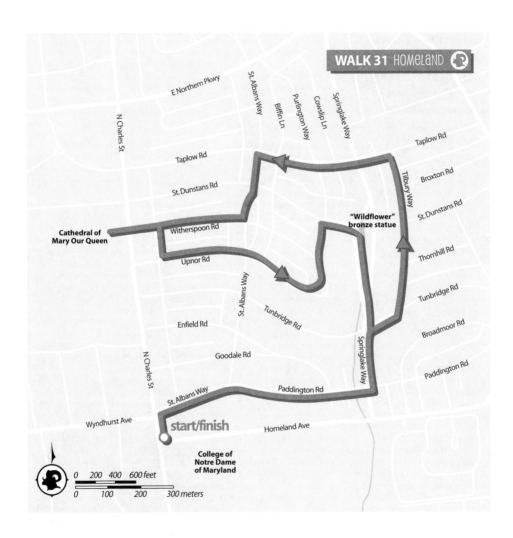

WALK 31 HOMELAND

E Northern Pkwy

St. Albans Way

Biffin Ln

Purlington Way

Cowslip Ln

Springlake Way

N Charles St

Taplow Rd

Taplow Rd

Broxton Rd

Tilbury Way

St. Dunstans Rd

St. Dunstans Rd

"Wildflower" bronze statue

Cathedral of
Mary Our Queen

Witherspoon Rd

Upnor Rd

Thornhill Rd

St. Albans Way

Tunbridge Rd

Tunbridge Rd

Enfield Rd

Broadmoor Rd

Goodale Rd

Springlake Way

Paddington Rd

N Charles St

Paddington Rd

St. Albans Way

Wyndhurst Ave

start/finish

Homeland Ave

College of
Notre Dame
of Maryland

0   200 400 600 feet

0   100   200   300 meters

31 HOMELAND: A NICE LAND TO CALL HOME

BOUNDARIES: **St. Albans Way, Paddington Rd., N. Charles St., Springlake Way, Taplow Rd.**
DISTANCE: **3 miles**
DIFFICULTY: **Moderate**
PARKING: **Street parking along entire route, with some residential restrictions**
PUBLIC TRANSIT: **MTA bus #11 runs along N. Charles St.**

This leafy and somewhat tony North Baltimore enclave was originally established in 1695 by Job Evans and was known as Job's Addition. Almost two centuries later, that tract of land, as well as neighboring tracts, had been purchased and maintained by David Maulden Perine. The almost-400-acre parcel, by then known as the Perine Estate of Homeland, became the neighborhood now known as Homeland. The Roland Park Company purchased it for $1 million (several of the houses there now would easily fetch that much and more) and turned it into one of the country's first planned communities in 1924. And the planning was sublimely done. As with other Roland Park Company planned neighborhoods (see Walk 29: Guilford and Walk 30: Roland Park), the terrain was incorporated into the design, a departure from earlier views of nature as something to subdue and form into more "human" lines and angles. In 2001, the entire neighborhood was entered into the National Register of Historic Places. Homeland's most well-known resident was novelist Anne Tyler (*The Accidental Tourist* is the most famous of her almost 20 novels), who lived here for several decades; Homeland lends itself as the setting of many of her books. It's no wonder she and so many others chose this wonderful urban neighborhood. A leisurely stroll through Homeland remains a pleasure, as it undoubtedly has for close to a hundred years now.

● On N. Charles St., just north of the campus of the College of Notre Dame of Maryland, across from the athletic complex for Loyola University, is Homeland Ave., the southern edge of Homeland. Go one block north to the more cozy St. Albans Way and head east, passing the white "Homeland 1924" sign.

The neighborhood's loveliness reveals itself immediately. This is simply a great urban enclave, with twisty, rolling streets; abundant plantings (it's a riot of azalea in spring); common green areas; mature trees; and an eclectic collection of architectural home styles using solid and stylish materials, with stucco, stone, and slate dominating. The majority of architectural styles you'll see walking around the neighborhood include: Colonial Revival, Dutch Colonial, Federal, Georgian Revival, and Tudor Revival.

- When St. Albans Way takes a sharp leftward turn, stay straight as the road becomes Paddington Rd. It might occur to you right away that the street names have a whiff of the English aristocracy about them. This is no coincidence. When the Roland Park Company first began to develop the area, they saw at once that the natural contours of the rolling terrain mimicked the English countryside they wished to emulate. Thus, they named the streets to match, as you'll notice throughout this walk.

- When you reach Springlake Way, take a left. You'll be in the 5100 block. Look for the house at 5108 Springlake Way; this was the first house approved by the Roland Park Company in 1924 and was built one year later.

- Take a right on Tunbridge Rd. This intersection, at Tunbridge Rd. and Springlake Way, is typical of so many Homeland intersections: four distinctive and beautiful houses facing each other at each corner.

- When the road splits, take a left onto Tilbury Way.

- Follow Tilbury Way for five blocks to Taplow Rd. and take a left. Following the route laid out in this description gives you a nice overview of the neighborhood and takes in a majority of it. But, as always, you are encouraged to trek off this route and check out side streets (if nothing else, Homeland has a series of service alleys that are among the nicest alleys you're likely to find anywhere).

- Follow Taplow Rd. west four blocks to St. Albans Way. After another block, just beyond St. Dunstans Rd., St. Albans Way splits, offering a nice ovoid green median anchored by a lovely bronzed cherub overlooking the intersection. Take the rightward curve and stay on St. Albans Way another block to a right onto Witherspoon Rd.

- Stay on Witherspoon Rd. until it ends at N. Charles St. You'll be directly across the street from the impressive Gothic Cathedral of Mary Our Queen. Local legend has it that Irish immigrant and wealthy merchant Thomas O'Neill ran downtown to survey his thriving dry-goods business at Charles and Lexington Sts. during the Great Fire of 1904. As O'Neill watched the fire roaring toward his business, he prayed that if his storefronts were spared, he would build a great cathedral out of gratitude. Sure enough, while the flames came close enough to lick at the south end of his business, the wind suddenly shifted the fire east and spared O'Neill's livelihood. O'Neill died in 1919 and after his wife followed him in 1936, the great bulk of his remaining fortune was left to make good on his promise. His will stipulated, "All the balance of my estate (including, after the death of my said sisters and brothers, the sum so as aforesaid put aside by my trustees to pay the annuities above mentioned) unto Most Reverend James Gibbons, Roman Catholic Archbishop of Baltimore . . . for the erecting of a Cathedral Church in the City of Baltimore." Go inside to check it out; it's an impressive place, complete with two stunning organs.

- When you are through at the cathedral, return to Witherspoon Rd. Take the first right through the service alley and follow it one block to a left onto Upnor Rd. Follow Upnor Rd. as it crosses St. Albans Way. At the corner of St. Albans Way and Upnor Rd. sits a private home that was once the Roland Park Company's caretaker's house, which functioned as the company's Homeland sales office.

- Follow Upnor Rd as it curves leftward toward Purlington Way. Purlington Way exists as a short semicircle stuck onto Upnor Rd. and then reemerges about 100 yards later along Upnor Rd. Take Purlington Way at this second meeting with Upnor Rd.

- Follow Purlington Way one block to a right onto St. Dunstans Rd. One block east is Springlake Way again. Here, it's absolutely exquisite. While calling this body of water in front of you a lake is something of a stretch, this pond and several others like it along Springlake Way exist as Homeland's finest natural (well,

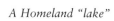

A Homeland "lake"

man-made) attractions. These six ponds, stocked with fish to help control mosquitoes, were dug in 1843, when the entire area was still part of David Perine's estate.
They froze over every winter to be enjoyed as skating rinks. Stone walls were added
near some of the ponds in 1960; the city undertook extensive renovation to these
walls and to each of the ponds in 1999 for the 75th anniversary of the neighborhood.
The ponds still have fish in them today, and with their fountains and plantings, they
give Homeland the aura of being an almost perfect urban neighborhood.

Make sure to check out the famous *Wildflower* bronze statue on the north side of
the middle lake on Springlake Way. A spritely girl with flower petals for hair, it has
become the unofficial image for Homeland. It was cast in 1909 by the Baltimore
sculptor and Maryland Institute alumnus Edward Berge, whose sculptures grace several Baltimore locations. Copies of *Wildflower* have been placed in parks all across
America. In 1915, Berge himself sent the bronze to the Panama Pacific Exposition in
San Francisco, and *Wildflower* was voted tops in show.

● Continue south on Springlake Way two blocks to Paddington Rd. Take a right and
head west to St. Albans Way to where you began this walk.

POINTS OF INTEREST (START TO FINISH)

Cathedral of Mary Our Queen cathedralofmary.org, 5200 N. Charles St., 410-464-4000

ROUTE SUMMARY

1. Start at St. Albans Way.
2. Go east on St. Albans Way until it turns into Paddington Rd.
3. Turn left onto Springlake Way.
4. Turn right onto Tunbridge Rd.
5. Turn left onto Tilbury Way.
6. Turn left onto Taplow Rd.
7. Turn left onto St. Albans Way.
8. Turn right onto Witherspoon Rd.
9. Cross N. Charles St. to visit the Cathedral of Mary Our Queen.

10.   Return to Witherspoon Rd.

11.   Turn right into the service alley parallel to Witherspoon Rd.

12.   Turn left onto Upnor Rd.

13.   Turn right onto Purlington Way.

14.   Turn right onto St. Dunstans Rd.

15.   Turn right onto Springlake Way.

16.   Turn right onto Paddington Rd.

17.   Follow Paddington Rd. to St. Albans Way.

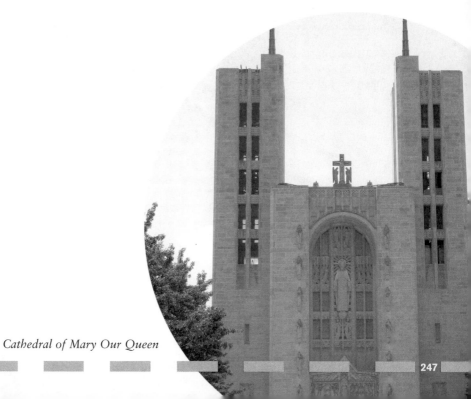

Cathedral of Mary Our Queen

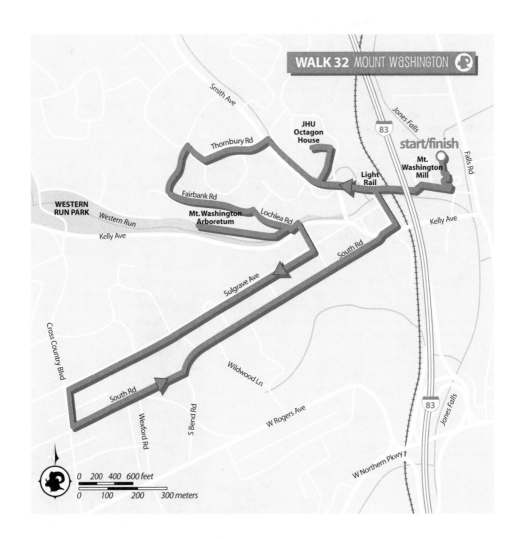

WALK 32 MOUNT WASHINGTON

Smith Ave

Thornbury Rd

JHU Octagon House

Jones Falls

83

start/finish

Light Rail

Mt. Washington Mill

Falls Rd

Fairbank Rd

WESTERN RUN PARK

Western Run

Mt. Washington Arboretum

Lochlea Rd

Kelly Ave

Kelly Ave

South Rd

Cross Country Blvd

Sulgrave Ave

Wildwood Ln

83

South Rd

Wexford Rd

S Bend Rd

W Rogers Ave

Jones Falls

W Northern Pkwy

0   200   400   600 feet
0   100   200   300 meters

32 MOUNT WASHINGTON: CITY CLOSE AND COUNTRY QUIET

BOUNDARIES: **Smith Ave., Greely Rd., Cross Country Blvd., South Rd.**
DISTANCE: **3.4 miles**
DIFFICULTY: **Moderate to strenuous**
PARKING: **At Mount Washington Mill and streets along route**
PUBLIC TRANSIT: **Mount Washington Light Rail; MTA bus #27 stops along Cross Country Blvd. and in Mount Washington Village. MTA buses #s 58, 60, and 61 all stop in Mount Washington Village.**

From its beginnings in the 1850s, Mount Washington was billed as a country place to escape the heat and grime of the city. With the advent of streetcars, Mount Washington became a place where one could do just that: enjoy the bucolic beauty and fresh air, but still be connected to downtown by the relatively short ride. H. L. Mencken's family was just one of Baltimore's many leading families who used to retreat to Mount Washington. (Even Al Capone, being treated at Union Memorial Hospital after his release from the Lewisburg Pen, got himself a house on Pimlico Road; ultimately, in a show of appreciation to the only hospital that would treat him, Capone planted a weeping cherry tree at the hospital, where it stands to this day. Only in Baltimore.) Walking around the tree-lined streets of Mount Washington, one is immediately struck by the obvious signs of community and neighborhood care. There is a palpable feeling here that the residents are all in on the same happy fantasy. Civility, tolerance, and diversity are buzzwords. The Mount Washington Improvement Association dates to 1885, making it one of the oldest such associations in the nation. It is as vigorous today as it has been for more than 125 years, and the signs of this are obvious all along this route.

● Begin at the Mt. Washington Mill complex. Hungry? Thirsty? There's a Starbucks, a Whole Foods Market, Sylvan Beach Ice Cream, the Mt. Washington Wine Company, and several other shops, all housed in a gorgeous 200-year-old refurbished cotton mill complex. Originally known as the Washington Cotton Factory, this mill complex began in 1807. Of the buildings you can see today, the oldest is the Stone Mill, from 1811. It originally operated as a water-powered cotton mill and is believed to be the third oldest of its kind surviving in the United States. But it's not just that the buildings in this complex have survived and are now tastefully reused; they are absolutely pristine and in remarkable shape. It's fun to simply wander among the warren of stone buildings while popping into the shops.

● When you've gotten your fill, literally and figuratively, walk toward the Jones Falls Expressway ramp (west of the mill complex) and head under it by taking the paved path to the other side of the JFX. This will take you to the Mount Washington Light Rail station. The exit road from the parking lot is Smith Ave. Take that heading west. Smith is named for a Yorkshire family who ran a dry-goods business nearby.

● Along Smith Ave., you'll almost immediately pass the Baltimore Clayworks, "a non-profit ceramic art center that exists to develop, sustain, and promote an artist-centered community that provides outstanding artistic, educational, and collaborative programs in ceramic arts." The Clayworks is housed on either side of the street in an 1880s stone house as well as an old library building.

● Pass Greely Rd. and take the path to the right heading down the hill. Soon you will come to an intersection with another path. Take it heading left toward the distinctive Octagon building. The Johns Hopkins University now owns this complex, but many locals remember it from when the USF&G insurance company was here. The Octagon dates to 1855 and spent its first six years of life as the Mt. Washington Female Seminary. The Catholic Order Sisters of Mercy bought the site and created the Mt. St. Agnes College before merging with Loyola College on Charles St. (Another octagonal building—this one a private home—appears later on this walk). The grounds are today quite lovely, and JHU rents out the facilities for private events.

● Head back to Smith Ave. and take a right, passing many attractive houses of varied architecture. Take your first left up Thornbury Rd. Straight ahead is the 1878 Mount Washington Presbyterian Church. This church, now the Chimes Senior Living Center, is an example of "stick" style construction, with machine-cut lumber, exposed wooden beams, and board-and-batten siding. It was a distinctly American style dating from the late 19th century. It has much in common with the more popular but later Queen Anne style.

● Continue up Thornbury, passing many beautiful Victorian houses, until you reach the confluence of Thornbury, Maywood Ave., and Dixon Rd. Where they meet you will find something of a local secret: a path heading through the woods to the left. Take it. You'll pop out on Fairbank Rd. When you reach Fairbank, take a left. Cape Cod–style houses line both sides of Fairbank initially, but eventually you'll see the same wonderful hodgepodge of architectural styles that helps to give Mt. Washington its uniqueness.

● When you reach Lochlea Rd., take a right and head down the hill. When you get to the bottom of the hill, just before you reach Kelly Ave., take a right into the Mount Washington Arboretum, a supremely cool 1-acre true oasis tucked into an unassuming corner of the neighborhood. Until 1989, there was an apartment complex here. That was flooded during Hurricane David and subsequently condemned and torn down. In its place came a showcase for native plants and shrubs. It is lovingly maintained and is free for anyone to come and wander and enjoy the beautiful solitude. In the decade-plus of its existence, it has served as a neighborhood meeting place, hosting solstice parties, Halloween celebrations, outdoor movies, and even a wedding or two. (Take note of the LOVE mural on the concrete retaining wall above the water near the far end of the arboretum.)

● After the arboretum, cross Kelly Ave. and take a right onto Sulgrave Ave., heading up the hill (be warned: it's a steep hill). Kelly Ave. was named for Simon Kelly, an Irish railroad employee working at the Mount Washington Station. He was so well known and well liked that riders climbing the hill up the road called it Kelly Ave. in his honor; when the neighborhood was annexed to Baltimore City years later, the name stuck. Sulgrave is a nod to the ancestral home of George Washington's family in Northamptonshire.

You'll immediately pass the locally beloved Mt. Washington Elementary. Across the street, at 1808 Sulgrave, is another octagonal house, this one built in 1885. This style of house was briefly popular in the United States in the mid-1800s; its popularity can be traced primarily to one man, phrenologist Orson Squire Fowler. These eight-sided houses became a fad because of their supposed ease for furnishing and maximal living space. Those that remain are usually oddities on the architectural scene, but their whimsical appearance rarely fails to draw curious—and often admiring—attention.

● Soon, at 1821 Sulgrave, you can see the house where great American author John Dos Passos (1896–1970) once lived. His U.S.A. trilogy made him famous and an admired contemporary of Hemingway, Fitzgerald, and others. Jean-Paul Sartre considered him "the greatest writer of our time." Dos Passos moved with his family to Baltimore in 1952. (Mount Washington wasn't his only Baltimore address; he also lived in Roland Park and Cross Keys, alongside another famous writer, Ogden Nash.)

● Sulgrave runs all the way to Mount Washington's busy western drag, Greenspring Ave. (quite beautiful in this area of the city), but it is ultimately up to you how far from the walk's starting point you want to go. My recommendation is to follow Sulgrave only as far as Cross Country Blvd. and make your way back. However, Mount Washington stretches far and wide, dipping all the way to Pimlico Race Track, home of the Preakness Stakes, the second jewel after the Kentucky Derby in horse racing's Triple Crown. Many of the side streets in this neighborhood beg for ambling. So take advantage of that. But to follow my specific instructions here, head to Cross Country Blvd., take a left, and then another left onto South Rd.

● If you followed the suggestion in the bullet point above, follow South Rd. all the way to Kelly Ave. As you walk this nice street, you will again see the varied but consistently lovely architecture of the houses that make up this unique neighborhood. So that you can keep yourself oriented, on the way to Kelly Ave. you will pass the following streets: Wexford Rd., Carterdale Rd., S. Bend Rd., Pollard St., Luddington St., Roxbury Pl., Helendale St., and Lochlea Rd. When you reach Kelly Ave. (to your left will be the St. John's Episcopal Church), cross Kelly Ave. and head left down the hill to rejoin Sulgrave and take a right. You are now in the heart of Mount Washington Village, a nice collection of shops and restaurants (including the venerable Mt. Washington Tavern, rebuilt after a 2011 fire, and the local favorites, Crepe du Jour and Ethel & Ramone's) and site of the annual Mount Washington Village Wine, Art & Jazz Festival, held each fall.

● Your starting point is easily reached by going left on Smith Ave. from Sulgrave, where you will see the Light Rail parking lot again.

POINTS OF INTEREST (START TO FINISH)

Mt. Washington Mill mtwashingtonmill.com, 1340 Smith Ave., 410-385-1234

Baltimore Clayworks baltimoreclayworks.org, 5707 Smith Ave., 410-578-1919

Octagon House acc-mtwashingtonconferencecenter.com, Mt. Washington Conference Center, 5801 Smith Ave., 800-488-8734

Mt. Washington Arboretum miniarboretum.org

Mount Washington Village mountwashingtonvillage.com

Mt. Washington Tavern mtwashingtontavern.com, 5700 Newbury St., 410-367-6903

Crepe du Jour crepedujour.com, 1609 Sulgrave Ave., 410-542-9000

Ethel & Ramone's ethelandramones.com, 1615 Sulgrave Ave., 410-664-2971

ROUTE SUMMARY

1. Start at Mt. Washington Mill.
2. Go under the JFX to Smith Ave. and head west.
3. Go right onto the path at the Mount Washington Conference Center to the Octagon House.
4. Return to Smith Ave. and go right.
5. Turn left onto Thornbury Rd.
6. Turn left onto the wooded path at the intersection of Thornbury, Maywood, and Dixon.
7. Emerge onto Fairbank Rd. and go left.
8. Turn right onto Lochlea Rd.
9. Turn right into the Mount Washington Arboretum.
10. Return to Lochlea and cross Kelly Ave.
11. Take a right onto Sulgrave Ave.
12. Turn left onto Cross Country Blvd.
13. Turn left onto South Rd.
14. Cross Kelly Ave. to take a right onto Sulgrave Rd.

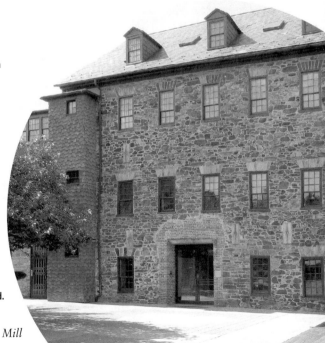

Mount Washington Mill

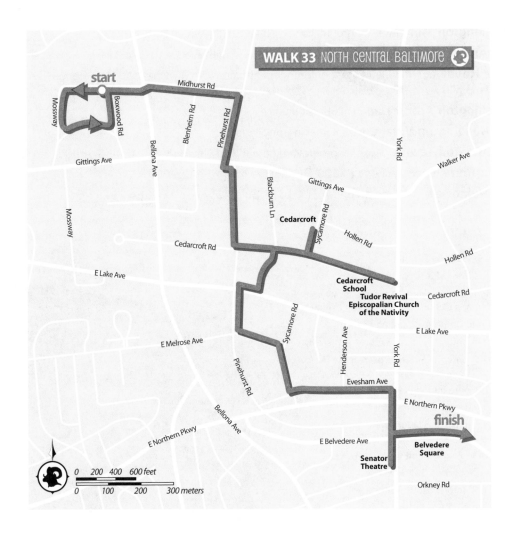

WALK 33 NORTH CENTRAL BALTIMORE

start

Midhurst Rd

Mossway

Boxwood Rd

Blenheim Rd

Pinehurst Rd

York Rd

Walker Ave

Gittings Ave

Gittings Ave

Bellona Ave

Mossway

Blackburn Ln

Cedarcroft

Sycamore Rd

Hollen Rd

Hollen Rd

Cedarcroft Rd

Cedarcroft
School
Tudor Revival
Episcopalian Church
of the Nativity

Cedarcroft Rd

E Lake Ave

E Lake Ave

E Melrose Ave

Sycamore Rd

Henderson Ave

York Rd

Pinehurst Rd

Evesham Ave

E Northern Pkwy

finish

Bellona Ave

E Northern Pkwy

E Belvedere Ave

Belvedere
Square

Senator
Theatre

Orkney Rd

0   200   400   600 feet
0   100   200   300 meters

33 NORTH CENTRAL BALTIMORE: WHO KNEW?

BOUNDARIES: **Midhurst Rd., Mossway, Pinehurst Rd., Sycamore Rd., Cedarcroft Rd., York Rd.**
DISTANCE: **3.3 miles**
DIFFICULTY: **Moderate**
PARKING: **All along route on residential streets**
PUBLIC TRANSIT: **MTA bus #11 runs along Bellona Ave.; MTA buses #8 and #12 run along York Rd. at Belvedere Square**

I'll admit it: I have a bias about the neighborhoods that comprise the northernmost stretches of central Baltimore city. These are the last pockets before you reach Baltimore County. They are wonderful neighborhoods—simply terrific places to live. I should know: it's where my wife and I bought our first house in Baltimore. And what I discovered then is what still largely holds true now: unless you live in these neighborhoods, you've probably never heard of them. I'm speaking of Pinehurst, Cedarcroft, Mossway, and Midhurst. They form the chain of neighborhoods abutting and sometimes spilling over the city line into the county, bordered to the south by Lake Evesham (better known and included here) and to the north by Rodgers Forge (better known still as the quintessential post-WWII town house neighborhood for returning vets). Compared to Baltimore County, the city takes some hits: after all, if you can live in Rodgers Forge, mere feet away from the city line and so close to everything the city has to offer, but pay half as much in property taxes, receive better and more efficient services, and enjoy blue ribbon schools, why would you choose to live in the city? There are plenty of easy answers to that one, of course. (This book provides a rather emphatic answer.) But the question is even more immediate when one chooses to live in one of these neighborhoods, so close to the advantages afforded by living in the county. Well, simply walk through these lovely places and you'll see the answer soon enough. Just don't give out the secret: remember, relatively few Baltimoreans even know these places exist. They may prove a surprise to you too—unless you live here, of course. And if you do, you already get it, don't you?

● **This book concentrates on city walks. That means that, technically, you'd have to limit yourself to staying south of the 6300 block of the north-south streets that straddle the city–county line here: Pinehurst Rd., Blenheim Rd., Bellona Ave., Boxwood Rd., and Mossway. Therefore, if you have a mind to be a stickler, you should begin this walk on Pinehurst Rd. south of 6300 (the numbers go in descending order as you** walk south into the city). My recommendation, however: be a rebel and slip into the county by starting at Midhurst Rd. just west of Bellona Ave. This is a lovely, leafy neighborhood—despite that, it's a nebulous sort of place: the mailing address is Baltimore, for lack of a better classification. It's definitely not Rodgers Forge and it doesn't quite make it to Cedarcroft or Bellona-Gittings, which are both city neighborhoods. I've heard it called Midhurst, Mossway, and even part of Pinehurst, though it's generally agreed that Pinehurst lies entirely on the east side of Bellona Ave.

Despite its "nowhere-ness," this little stretch of homes and mature trees is gorgeous. This short diversion acts as a pleasant add-on to the walk proper. To do it right, then (and not worry so much about trifling distinctions such as city–county lines), take Midhurst Rd. west as it swings leftward and becomes Mossway. This street is where accomplished author, *Sports Illustrated* columnist, and National Public Radio contributor Frank DeFord grew up.

- Take a left from Mossway onto Thicket Rd. Here you could spit into the city; the line is mere feet in front of you. But stay in the county for now by taking the semicircular Thicket Rd. until you shortly reach Boxwood Rd. and take a left. Follow Boxwood Rd. back to Midhurst Rd., where you began.

- This time, head east on Midhurst Rd. and cross Bellona Ave., taking in the lovely houses around you. This is what residential suburbia should be: solid, attractive, and varied housing; mature trees; and close proximity to amenities. The evidence that this is a wonderful place to raise kids will be all around you: a proliferation of lacrosse nets, bicycles, basketball hoops, and all the detritus of childhoods well spent.

- When you reach Pinehurst Rd., take a right. You'll very soon cross into the city, but no official signage tells you so. You will, however, soon see some Cedarcroft signs.

- When you reach Gittings Ln., cross it to stay on Pinehurst Rd. Here, the street narrows; a royal assemblage of towering sycamores lines the street on both sides. You'll soon reach Cedarcroft Rd. This is a particularly lovely intersection: a glance down either side of Cedarcroft Rd. from Pinehurst Rd. reveals many examples of the wonderfully varied architecture: American Foursquare, Bungalow, Cape Cod, Dutch Colonial, Federal, Georgian, Italianate, Spanish Colonial.

- From Pinehurst Rd., take a left onto Cedarcroft Rd. Pass Blackburn Ln. and take a left onto Sycamore Rd. Just a bit up Sycamore Rd. on the left is a house at #6204, built by Philip Lamb in 1886. This house, along with the 46 acres Lamb purchased, comprised his estate, Cedarcroft. The Cedarcroft Land Company began in 1910, as did construction on the houses you see all around you.

- Return to Cedarcroft Rd. and take a left. Up the road to the right, at 419 Cedarcroft Rd., is the Cedarcroft School, a preschool founded in 1947 that is deeply woven into the fabric of the community. The building where the school resides was originally built in 1923 as a parish house for the adjoining church, and it's a gorgeous example of Gothic Revival architecture. Just beyond it, paralleling busy York Rd., is the Tudor Revival Episcopalian Church of the Nativity, originally built in western Maryland, dismantled, and then moved to its present location for services beginning in 1913.

- To avoid busy York Rd., turn around and return down Cedarcroft Rd. until you reach Blackburn Ln. and take a left. Blackburn Ln. is a wonderful example of what happens when city planners work with nature instead of against it. Again, towering trees dominate, but gone are the long, straight shots of Pinehurst Rd. and Cedarcroft Rd. Blackburn Ln. is a windy, narrow little street.

- When you reach the broad E. Lake Ave., take a right. Pinehurst Rd. is just up the street. Take a left onto Pinehurst Rd.

  Here, Pinehurst Rd. takes a more modest turn. The houses and the neighborhood are still lovely. But these houses are mostly brick-and-siding porch-front homes, with many frame cottages scattered about. You're now entering the neighborhood of Lake Evesham (don't look for a lake; there isn't one). This area was once part of the 1877 estate of Samuel Brady called Midwood. The largest parcel of that divided estate, Chestnut Park, makes up today's Lake Evesham.

- Take a left on E. Melrose Ave. At the end of the road, take a right onto Sycamore Rd. Follow Sycamore Rd. to a left onto Evesham Ave. You'll be paralleling the busy E. Northern Pkwy. Turn right at York Rd., taking great care by crossing E. Northern Pkwy. at the light. You're now in a different world. But it's a pretty cool one: shops, restaurants, and the wonderfully revitalized Belvedere Square a few hundred yards to the left. But before you make a beeline for Belvedere Square, make sure to check out the Senator Theatre, added to the National Register of Historic Places in 1989, on the west side of York Rd., across from Belvedere Square. The Senator enjoys a rich history in Baltimore. Built in 1939, this Art Deco one-screen movie house is one of just a few of its kind left in the country. Outside, you'll see a walk of fame, complete with handprint impresses and celebrations of past premieres. Baltimore natives and filmmakers Barry Levinson and John Waters often premiere their movies at the Senator, and many top-flight stars appear for movies shot in Baltimore (John Travolta and Joaquin Phoenix for *Ladder 49,* for example) or because they are native to the area (Edward Norton, Josh Charles, and Jada Pinkett Smith, for example). Even if you don't watch a film, the lobby is worth checking out. The floors are original terrazzo, and Art Deco murals grace the walls. In recent years, the Senator's future was in question, but interventions and financial aid from the city as well as new ownership has meant that the Senator will, for the foreseeable future at least, remain one of Baltimore's unique historic (and still-functioning) jewels. *Note:* The Senator underwent renovations in 2012; check its website for progress.

- Across York Rd. from the Senator Theatre is Belvedere Square. The mix of shops, restaurants, and services that comprise Belvedere Square opened in 1986 and immediately became a draw for the then-somewhat-neglected area of north Baltimore. Many area residents remember how quickly it reverted into something of a no-go zone. One by one the shops closed up, and a feud between the developer and local residents resulted in Belvedere Square turning into a wasteland by the mid-1990s. But by 2000, new developers, city partnerships, and input from the local community not only returned Belvedere Square to its former glory, but exceeded it. It's now a wonderful place to visit to enjoy wine, fresh and local produce from area farms, restaurants, and upscale shopping. Summer concerts turn Belvedere Square into the community gathering place it was originally envisioned to be.

- There are several ways to return to your starting point at Bellona Ave. and Midhurst Rd. Of course, you can retrace your steps. But if you prefer to go by foot on a slightly different route, you can walk north up York Rd. to any one of three east–west roads, all on the left: E. Lake Ave., Cedarcroft Rd., and Gittings Ave. All three will intersect with Bellona Ave., where you will take a right to reach Midhurst Rd. Alternately, if you wish to take public transportation, go back to E. Northern Pkwy., catch an MTA bus heading west, and get off at the next stop at Bellona Ave. There, pick up the #11 to Towson, which stops at Bellona Ave. and Midhurst Rd., your starting point.

POINTS OF INTEREST (START TO FINISH)

Cedarcroft School cedarcroftschool.com, 419 Cedarcroft Rd., 410-435-0905

Church of the Nativity nativitycedarcroft.org, 419 Cedarcroft Rd., 410-433-4811

Senator Theatre thesenatortheatre.com, 5904 York Rd., 410-323-4665

Belvedere Square belvederesquare.com, 518 E. Belvedere Ave., 410-464-9773

ROUTE SUMMARY

1. Start at Midhurst Rd., just west of Bellona Ave.
2. Follow Midhurst Rd. west as it turns into Mossway.
3. Turn left onto Thicket Rd.
4. Turn left onto Boxwood Rd.
5. Turn right onto Midhurst Rd.
6. Cross Bellona Ave. on Midhurst Rd. and take a right onto Pinehurst Rd.
7. Take a left onto Cedarcroft Rd.
8. Take a left onto Sycamore Rd. to 6204 Sycamore Rd.
9. Return to Cedarcroft Rd. and take a left to 419 Cedarcroft Rd.
10. Reverse direction on Cedarcroft Rd. and take a left onto Blackburn Ln.
11. Take a right onto E. Lake Ave.
12. Take a left onto Pinehurst Rd.
13. Take a left onto E. Melrose Ave.
14. Take a right onto Sycamore Rd.
15. Take a left onto Evesham Ave.
16. Cross E. Northern Pkwy.
17. Go south on York Rd. to the Senator Theatre and Belvedere Square.

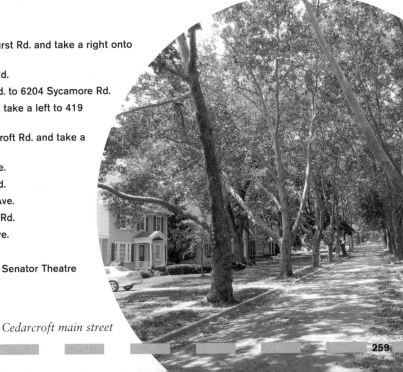

Cedarcroft main street

Appendix 1: WaLKS BY THeMe

american FirSTS

Fort McHenry (Walk 1)
Inner Harbor Promenade (Walk 4)
Fells Point (Walk 6)
Canton & Brewers Hill (Walk 7)
Little Italy & Jonestown/Old Town (Walk 10)
Civil War Trail (Walk 11)
Downtown: Contrasts (Walk 12)
SOWEBO (Walk 14)
Mount Vernon (Walk 16)
Pennsylvania Avenue (Walk 17)
Seton Hill & Lexington Market (Walk 18)
Mount Royal (Walk 20)
Charles Village & JHU (Walk 25)
Hampden & Wyman Park (Walk 27)
Roland Park (Walk 30)

Green SpaceS

Fort McHenry (Walk 1)
Gwynns Falls Trail II: Westport Waterfront
(Walk 2)
Federal Hill (Walk 3)
Patterson Park to Highlandtown (Walk 9)
Gwynns Falls Trail: From Leon Day to
Mount Clare (Walk 15)
Mount Vernon (Walk 16)

Falls Road Turnpike (Walk 22)
Druid Hill Park (Walk 23)
Dickeyville & Leakin Park (Walk 24)
Lake Montebello & Herring Run (Walk 26)
Hampden & Wyman Park (Walk 27)
Guilford (Walk 29)

ICONIC BaLTiMOre

Fort McHenry (Walk 1)
Federal Hill (Walk 3)
Inner Harbor Promenade (Walk 4)
Fells Point (Walk 6)
Canton & Brewers Hill (Walk 7)
Patterson Park to Highlandtown (Walk 9)
Little Italy & Jonestown/Old Town (Walk 10)
Downtown: The Raven to the Ravens (Walk 13)
SOWEBO (Walk 14)
Mount Vernon (Walk 16)
Charles Village & JHU (Walk 25)
Hampden & Wyman Park (Walk 27)

THe MONUMeNTaL CiTY

Fort McHenry (Walk 1)
Federal Hill (Walk 3)
Inner Harbor Promenade (Walk 4)
Harbor East (Walk 5)

Fells Point (Walk 6)
Canton & Brewers Hill (Walk 7)
Patterson Park to Highlandtown (Walk 9)
Civil War Trail (Walk 11)
Downtown: Contrasts (Walk 12)
Downtown: The Raven to the Ravens (Walk 13)
Mount Vernon (Walk 16)
Pennsylvania Avenue (Walk 17)
Seton Hill & Lexington Market (Walk 18)
Bolton Hill (Walk 19)
Mount Royal (Walk 20)
Druid Hill Park (Walk 23)
Lake Montebello & Herring Run (Walk 26)
Guilford (Walk 29)

MUSEUM MADNESS

Fort McHenry (Walk 1)
Federal Hill (Walk 3)
Inner Harbor Promenade (Walk 4)
Harbor East (Walk 5)
Fells Point (Walk 6)
Little Italy & Jonestown/Old Town (Walk 10)
Civil War Trail (Walk 11)
Downtown: The Raven to the Ravens (Walk 13)
SOWEBO (Walk 14)
Gwynns Falls Trail: From Leon Day to Mount
    Clare (Walk 15)
Mount Vernon (Walk 16)
Seton Hill & Lexington Market (Walk 18)
Falls Road Turnpike (Walk 22)
Charles Village & JHU (Walk 25)
Guilford (Walk 29)

WATERFRONT

Fort McHenry (Walk 1)
Gwynns Falls Trail II: Westport Waterfront
    (Walk 2)
Inner Harbor Promenade (Walk 4)
Harbor East (Walk 5)
Fells Point (Walk 6)
Canton & Brewers Hill (Walk 7)
Gwynns Falls Trail: From Leon Day to
    Mount Clare (Walk 15)
Falls Road Turnpike (Walk 22)
Lake Montebello & Herring Run (Walk 26)

WRITERS & READERS

Fells Point (Walk 6)
Canton & Brewers Hill (Walk 7)
Patterson Park to Highlandtown (Walk 9)
Downtown: Contrasts (Walk 12)
Downtown: The Raven to the Ravens (Walk 13)
SOWEBO (Walk 14)
Mount Vernon (Walk 16)
Bolton Hill (Walk 19)
Mount Royal (Walk 20)
Dickeyville & Leakin Park (Walk 24)
Charles Village & JHU (Walk 25)
Hampden & Wyman Park (Walk 27)
Guilford (Walk 29)
Roland Park (Walk 30)
Homeland (Walk 31)
Mount Washington (Walk 32)

Appendix 2: POINTS OF INTEREST

Bars & Restaurants

Acropolis acropolisbaltimore.com, 4718 Eastern Ave., 410-675-3384 (Walk 8)

Alewife alewifebaltimore.com, 21 N. Eutaw St., 410-545-5112 (Walk 13)

Atman's Delicatessen atmansdeli.com, 1019 E. Lombard St., 410-563-2666 (Walk 10)

Bo Brooks bobrooks.com, 2701 Boston St., 410-558-0202 (Walk 7)

The Brewer's Art brewersart.com, 1106 N. Charles St., 410-547-6925 (Walk 16)

Café Hon cafehon.com, 1002 W. 36th St., 410-243-1230 (Walk 27)

Charleston charlestonrestaurant.com, 1000 Lancaster St., 410-332-7373 (Walk 5)

Ciao Bella cbella.com, 236 S. High St., 410-685-7733 (Walk 10)

Cinghiale cgeno.com, 822 Lancaster St., 410-547-8282 (Walk 5)

Claddagh Pub claddaghonline.com, 2918 O'Donnell St., 410-522-4220 (Walk 7)

Club Charles 1724 N. Charles St., 410-727-8815 (Walk 21)

Crêpe Du Jour crepedujour.com, 1609 Sulgrave Ave., 410-542-9000 (Walk 32)

Darker Than Blue Café darkerthanbluecafe.com, 3034 Greenmount Ave., 443-872-4468 (Walk 25)

DiPasquale's Marketplace dipasquales.com, 3700 Gough St., 410-276-6787 (Walk 9)

Dogwood dogwoodbaltimore.com, 911 W. 36th St., 410-889-0952 (Walk 27)

Ethel & Ramone's ethelandramones.com, 1615 Sulgrave Ave., 410-664-2971 (Walk 32)

Golden West Café goldenwestcafe.com, 1105 W. 36th St., 410-889-8891 (Walk 27)

Grano Emporio granopastabar.com, 3547 Chestnut Ave., 443-438-7521 (Walk 27)

Grano Pasta Bar granopastabar.com, 1031 W. 36th St., 443-869-3429 (Walk 27)

The Helmand helmand.com, 806 N. Charles St., 410-752-0311 (Walk 16)

Hoehn's Bakery hoehnsbakery.com, 400 S. Conkling St., 410-675-2884 (Walk 9)

Holy Frijoles holyfrijoles.net, 908 W. 36th St., 410-235-2326 (Walk 27)

The Horse You Came In On thehorsebaltimore.com, 1626 Thames St., 410-327-8111 (Walk 6)

Ikaros ikarosrestaurant.com, 4805 Eastern Ave., 410-633-3750 (Walk 8)

James Joyce Pub jamesjoycepub.com, 616 S. President St., 410-727-5107 (Walk 5)

Joe Squared 133 W. North Ave., 410-545-0444, joesquared.com (Walk 21)

Lebanese Taverna lebanesetaverna.com, 719 S. President St., 410-244-5533 (Walk 5)

Matthew's Pizzeria matthewspizza.com, 3131 Eastern Ave., 410-276-8755 (Walk 9)

Mick O'Shea's mickosheas.com, 328 N. Charles St., 410-539-7504 (Walk 16)

Miss Shirley's Café missshirleyscafe.com, 750 E. Pratt St., 410-528-5373 (Walk 11)

Mt. Washington Tavern mtwashingtontavern.com, 5700 Newbury St., 410-367-6903 (Walk 32)

One World Café one-world-café.com, 100 W. University Pkwy., 410-235-5777 (Walk 25)

Petit Louis petitlouis.com, 4800 Roland Ave., 410-366-9393 (Walk 30)

The Rusty Scupper selectrestaurants.com/rusty, 402 Key Hwy., 410-727-3678 (Walk 4)

Sabatino's sabatinos.com, 901 Fawn St., 410-727-9414 (Walk 10)

Sammy's Trattoria sammystrattoria.com, 1200 N. Charles St., 410-837-9999 (Walk 20)

Samos samosrestaurant.com, 600 Oldham St., 410-675-5292 (Walk 8)

Sofi's Crepes sofiscrepes.com, 1723 N. Charles St., 410-727-7732 (Walk 21)

Tapas Teatro tapasteatro.com, 1711 N. Charles St., 410-332-0110 (Walk 21)

Tio Pepe tiopepebaltimore.com, 10 E. Franklin St., 443-863-8808 (Walk 16)

Waterfront Hotel waterfronthotel.us, 1710 Thames St., 410-537-5055 (Walk 6)

The Windup Space thewindupspace.com, 12 W. North Ave., 410-244-8855 (Walk 21)

Woodberry Kitchen woodberrykitchen.com, 2010 Clipper Park Rd. #126, 410-464-8000 (Walk 28)

Colleges, Universities, & Bookstores

Atomic Books atomicbooks.com, 3620 Falls Rd., 410-662-4444 (Walk 27)

The Book Thing of Baltimore bookthing.org, 3001 Vineyard Ln., 410-662-5631 (Walk 25)

The Johns Hopkins University jhu.edu, 3400 N. Charles St. (Walk 25)

Loyola University of Maryland loyola.edu, 4501 N. Charles St., 410-617-2000 or 800-221-9107 (Walk 29)

Maryland Institute College of Art mica.edu, 1300 W. Mount Royal Ave., 410-669-9200 (Walk 20)

Normal's Bookstore normals.com, 425 E. 31st St., 410-243-6888 (Walk 25)

University of Baltimore ubalt.edu, 1420 N. Charles St., 410-837-4200 (Walk 20)

University of Maryland at Baltimore umaryland.edu, 620 W. Lexington St. (Walk 13)

cultural attractions

Baltimore Visitor Center baltimore.org, 401 Light St., 877-BALTIMORE (Walk 4)

Baltimore Symphony Orchestra/Meyerhoff Symphony Hall bsomusic.org, 1212 Cathedral St., 410-783-8000 (Walk 20)

Carrie Murray Nature Center carriemurraynaturecenter.org, 1901 Ridgetop Rd., 410-396-0808 (Walk 24)

Enoch Pratt Free Library, Canton Branch prattlibrary.org, 1030 S. Ellwood Ave., 410-545-7130 (Walk 7)

Enoch Pratt Free Library, Central Branch prattlibrary.org, 400 Cathedral St., 410-396-5430 (Walk 16)

Enoch Pratt Free Library, Roland Park Branch prattlibrary.org, 5108 Roland Ave. (Walk 30)

Enoch Pratt Free Library, Southeast Anchor Branch prattlibrary.org, 3601 Eastern Ave., 410-396-1580 (Walk 9)

Eubie Blake National Jazz Institute and Cultural Center eubieblake.org, 847 N. Howard St., 410-225-3130 (Walk 16)

France-Merrick Performing Arts Center/Hippodrome Theatre france-merrickpac.com, 12 N. Eutaw St., 410-837-7400 (Walk 13)

Hollywood Diner 400 E. Saratoga St. (Walk 12)

Lyric Opera House lyricoperahouse.com, 110 W. Mount Royal Ave., 410-685-5086 (Walk 20)

Maryland Historical Society mdhs.org, 201 W. Monument St., 410-685-3750 (Walk 16)

Maryland Science Center mdsci.org, 601 Light St., 410-685-5225 (Walk 4)

Maryland Zoo in Baltimore marylandzoo.org, Druid Hill Park, 410-396-7102 (Walk 23)

Miracle on 34th Street 700 block of W. 34th St. (Walk 27)

National Aquarium in Baltimore aqua.org, 501 E. Pratt St., 410-576-3800 (Walk 4)

National Pinball Museum nationalpinballmuseum.org, 608 Water St., 443-438-1241 (Walk 5)

Plateia 700 block of S. Ponca St. (Walk 8)

Port Discovery Children's Museum portdiscovery.org, 35 Market Pl., 410-727-8120 (Walk 5)

Power Plant Live! powerplantlive.com, 34 Market Pl., 410-752-5483 (Walk 5)

Rawlings Conservatory rawlingsconservatory.org, 3100 Swann Dr., 410-396-0008, (Walk 23)

Senator Theatre thesenatortheatre.com, 5904 York Rd., 410-323-4665 (Walk 33)

Star-Spangled Banner Flag House flaghouse.org, 844 E. Pratt St., 410-837-1793 (Walk 10)

The Vagabond Theatre vagabondplayers.org, 806 S. Broadway, 410-563-9135 (Walk 6)

World Trade Center Observation Level viewbaltimore.org, 401 E. Pratt St., 27th floor, 410-837-VIEW (Walk 4, Walk 11)

Historic Markets

Avenue Market 1700 Pennsylvania Ave. (Walk 17)

Broadway Market 600 and 700 blocks of S. Broadway (Walk 6)

Cross Street Market Cross St. between Light and Charles Sts. (Walk 3)

Hollins Market 26 S. Arlington Ave., 410-685-6169 (Walk 14)

Lexington Market lexingtonmarket.com, 400 W. Lexington St., 410-685-6169 (Walk 13, Walk 18)

Historic Religious Institutions

The Baltimore Basilica baltimorebasilica.org, 409 Cathedral St., 410-727-3565 (Walk 16)

Baltimore Masjid 514 Islamic Way (Walk 17)

Brown Memorial Presbyterian Church 1316 Park Ave., 410-523-1542 (Walk 19)

Cathedral of Mary Our Queen cathedralofmary.org, 5200 N. Charles St., 410-464-4000 (Walk 31)

Church of the Nativity nativitycedarcroft.org, 419 Cedarcroft Rd., 410-433-4811 (Walk 33)

Eutaw Place Temple 1307 Eutaw Pl. (Walk 19)

Eutaw Place Baptist Church Dolphin and Eutaw Sts. (Walk 19)

First Unitarian Church of Baltimore 12 W. Franklin St., 410-685-2330 (Walk 16)

Greek Orthodox Cathedral of the Annunciation goannun.org, 24 W. Preston St., 410-727-2641 (Walk 20)

Mount Vernon Place United Methodist Church 10 E. Mt. Vernon Pl. (Walk 16)

Old Otterbein United Methodist Church oldotterbeinumc.org, 112 W. Conway St., 410-685-4703 (Walk 11)

Roland Park Presbyterian Church 4801 Roland Ave. (Walk 30)

Sailor's Union Bethel Methodist Church 454 E. Cross St. (Walk 3)

St. Jude Shrine stjudeshrine.org, 512 W. Saratoga St., 410-685-6026 (Walk 18)

Saint Nicholas Greek Orthodox Church 520 S. Ponca St., 410-633-5020 (Walk 8)

St. Patrick's Roman Catholic Church Broadway and Bank St. (Walk 6)

Saint Peter Claver Roman Catholic Church 1546 N. Fremont Ave. (Walk 17)

St. Michael The Archangel Ukrainian Catholic Church 2401 Eastern Ave. (Walk 9)

St. Stanislaus Kostka Roman Catholic Church Aliceanna and S. Ann Sts. (Walk 6)

Trinity Baptist Church 1600 Druid Hill Ave. (Walk 17)

Zion Lutheran Church zionbaltimore.org, 400 E. Lexington St., 410-727-3939 (Walk 12)

Historic Sites

Admiral Fell Inn harbormagic.com, 888 S. Broadway, 410-539-2000 (Walk 6)

Belt's Wharf 936 Fell St. (Walk 6)

Broadway Pier Broadway and Thames St. (Walk 6)

Brown's Wharf Broadway and Thames St. (Walk 6)

Captain John Steele House 931 Fell St. (Walk 6)

City Recreation Pier 1700 block of Thames St. (Walk 6)

Crown Cork & Seal Plant Eastern Ave. (Walk 8)

Douglass Terrace Dallas St. (Walk 6)

Fell Family Grave Marker 1607 Shakespeare St. (Walk 6)

Fort McHenry National Monument and Historic Shrine 2400 E. Fort Ave. (Walk 1)

George Wells House/London Coffee House Northwest corner of Bond and Thames Sts./ 854 S. Bond St. (Walk 6)

Greenmount Cemetery greenmountcemetary.com, 1501 Greenmount Ave., 410-539-0641 (Walk 21)

Henderson's Wharf Fell and Wolfe Sts. (Walk 6)

Historic Ships in Baltimore historicships.org, Pier 1, 301 E. Pratt St., 410-5391797: **USS *Constellation***: historicships.org/constellation; **USCGC *Taney***: historicships.org/taney; **USS *Torsk***: historicships.org/torsk; **LV116 *Chesapeake***: historicships.org/chesapeake; **Seven Foot Knoll Lighthouse**: historicships.org/knoll-lighthouse (Walk 4)

The Horse You Came In On thehorsebaltimore.com, 1626 Thames St., 410-327-8111 (Walk 6)

Merchant's House 1732 Thames St. (Walk 6)

Mount Royal Station www.mica.edu/browse_art/mount_royal_station.html, 1300 W. Mount Royal Ave., 410-669-9200 (Walk 20)

Mt. Vernon Mill complex millno1.com, 3000 Falls Rd., 410-327-3200 (Walk 22)

Orianda House/Crimea Estate friendsoforiandahouse.com, Leakin Park, 1901 Eagle Dr., 410-299-7613 (Walk 24)

Peale Museum 225 N. Holliday St. (Walk 12)

Robert Long House 812 S. Ann St. / **Society for the Preservation of Federal Hill and Fells Point** preservationsociety.com, 410-675-6750 (Walk 6)

St. Mary's Spritual Center & Historic Site/Mother Seton House stmarysspiritualcenter.org / mothersetonhouse.org; 600 North Paca St.; 410-728-6464 (central office) / 410-523-3443 (Mother Seton House) (Walk 18)

Saint Paul's Lutheran Cemetery Druid Hill Park (Walk 23)

Seaman's Hall 802 S. Broadway (Walk 6)

Swann's Wharf 1001 Fell St. (Walk 6)

Tavern/Sweatshop 1738 Thames St. (Walk 6)

Thurgood Marshall Childhood Home 1632 Division St. (Walk 17)

William Price House 910 Fell St. (Walk 6)

Wooden Houses 612–614 Wolfe St. (Walk 6)

YMCA 1609 Druid Hill Ave. (Walk 17)

MONUMENTS & MEMORIALS

9/11 Memorial World Trade Center, 401 E. Pratt St. (Walk 4, Walk 11)

Babe Ruth Statue S. Eutaw and W. Camden Sts. (Walk 13)

Barye Lion Mount Vernon Pl. (Walk 16)

Battle Monument Calvert St., between Fayette St. and Lexington St. (Walk 12)

Billie Holiday Plaza 1386 Pennsylvania Ave. at W. Lafayette Ave. (Walk 17)

Black Soldiers Statue 100 N. Holliday St. (Walk 12)

Boy Scout Statue Boy Scout Park, Sisson St. and Wyman Park Dr. (Walk 22)

Brooks Robinson Statue Washington Blvd. and W. Camden St. (Walk 13)

Cal Ripken Jr. Statue Washington Blvd. and W. Camden St. (Walk 13)

Casimir Pulaski Monument pattersonpark.com, Patterson Park, 27 S. Patterson Park Ave., 410-276-3676 (Walk 9)

Cecilius Calvert Statue E. Lexington St. and Saint Paul St. (Walk 12)

Christopher Columbus Monument Columbus Park, Eastern Ave., S. President St., Fawn St., and E. Falls Ave. (Walk 4)

Christopher Columbus Monument druidhillpark.org, Druid Hill Park (Walk 23)

Christopher Columbus Obelisk Harford Rd. and Walther Ave. (Walk 26)

Conradin Kreutzer Monument pattersonpark.com, Patterson Park, 27 S. Patterson Park Ave. (Walk 9)

Creators' Game Statue Lacrosse Hall of Fame, Johns Hopkins University, 113 W. University Pkwy. (Walk 25)

Daniel Coit Gilman Statue Johns Hopkins University, Shriver Hall (Walk 25)

Earl Weaver Statue Washington Blvd. and W. Camden St. (Walk 13)

Eddie Murray Statue Washington Blvd. and W. Camden St. (Walk 13)

Edgar Allan Poe Memorial (Cemetery) westminsterhall.org, Westminster Hall, 519 W. Fayette St., 410-706-2072 (Walk 13)

Edgar Allan Poe Statue W. Mount Royal and Maryland Aves., University of Baltimore (Walk 20)

Eli Siegel Monument druidhillpark.org, Druid Hill Park, 443-469-8274 (Walk 23)

Firefighters' Memorial N. Gay and Lexington Sts. (Walk 12)

Francis Scott Key Mount Vernon Place United Methodist Church mvp-umc.org, 10 E. Mt. Vernon Pl. (Walk 16)

Francis Scott Key Memorial Eutaw Pl. and W. Lanvale St. (Walk 19)

Frank Robinson Statue Washington Blvd. and W. Camden St. (Walk 13)

Frank Zappa Monument Enoch Pratt Free Library, Southeast Anchor Branch, 3601 Eastern Ave., 410-396-1580 (Walk 9)

Frederick Douglass Bust S. Caroline and Philpot Sts. (Walk 6)

George Armistead Monument Fort McHenry National Monument and Historic Shrine nps.gov/fomc, 2400 E. Fort Ave., 410-962-4290 (Walk 1)

George Armistead Monument Federal Hill Park, Battery and Warren Aves. (Walk 3)

George Washington Washington Monument and Museum at Mount Vernon Place, 699 N. Charles St., 410-396-1049 (Walk 16)

George Washington druidhillpark.org, Druid Hill Park, 443-469-8274 (Walk 23)

Hanover Street/Vietnam Veterans Memorial Bridge Hanover St. (Walk 2)

Holocaust Memorial E. Lombard and S. Gay Sts. (Walk 12)

Isaiah Bowman Bust Johns Hopkins University, Shriver Hall (Walk 25)

Jim Palmer Statue Washington Blvd. and W. Camden St. (Walk 13)

John Cook Memorial Rose Garden Sundial druidhillpark.org, Druid Hill Park, 3100 Swann Dr., 443-469-8274 (Walk 23)

John Eager Howard Statue Mount Vernon Pl. (Walk 16)

John O'Donnell Statue O'Donnell and S. Curley Sts. (Walk 7)

Johnny Unitas Statue S. Eutaw and W. Camden Sts. (Walk 13)

Jose Marti Bust N. Broadway and E. Fayette St. (Walk 6)

Katyn Massacre Memorial katynbaltimore.com, S. President St. Roundabout (Walk 5)

Korean War Memorial Canton Waterfront Park, 2903 Boston St. (Walk 7)

Marquis de Lafayette Statue Mount Vernon Pl. (Walk 16)

Martin Luther Statue Hillen Rd. and E. 32nd St. (Walk 26)

Maryland Line Monument Cathedral St. and W. Mount Royal Ave. (Walk 20)

Memorial Stadium Urn S. Eutaw and W. Lee Sts. (Walk 13)

Military Courage Statue Mount Vernon Pl. (Walk 16)

Northeast District Memorial to Fallen Officers Harford Rd. and Parkside Dr. (Walk 26)

Orpheus (Francis Scott Key) Fort McHenry National Monument and Historic Shrine, 2400 E. Fort Ave. (Walk 1)

Pool No. 2 Monument Druid Hill Park (Walk 23)

Richard Wagner Bust druidhillpark.org, Druid Hill Park, Lake Dr., 443-469-8274 (Walk 23)

Rodgers' Bastion Memorial Cannon pattersonpark.com, Patterson Park, E. Pratt St. and S. Patterson Park Ave., 410-276-3676 (Walk 9)

Roger Brooke Taney Statue Mount Vernon Pl. (Walk 16)

Royal Marquee Monument Pennsylvania and W. Lafayette Aves. (Walk 17)

Samuel Smith Monument Federal Hill Park, Battery and Warren Aves. (Walk 3)

Severn Teackle Wallis Statue Mount Vernon Pl. (Walk 16)

Sidney Lanier Statue Johns Hopkins University, 3436 N. Charles St. (Walk 25)

Simon Bolivar Bust N. Charles St., St Paul St., and Bedford Pl. (Walk 29)

Spirit of the Confederacy Monument Mount Royal Terr. between Mosher St. and Lafayette (Walk 20)

Star-Spangled Banner Centennial Monument pattersonpark.com, Patterson Park, E. Pratt St. and S. Patterson Park Ave., 410-276-3676 (Walk 9)

Thomas Wildey Odd Fellows Monument N. Broadway and E. Fayette St. (Walk 6)

Thurgood Marshall Statue Hopkins Pl. and W. Pratt St. (Walk 11)

War Memorial 101 N. Gay St., 410-396-8013 (Walk 12)

William Donald Schaefer Statue Light and E. Conway Sts. (Walk 4)

William Wallace Statue druidhillpark.org, Druid Hill Park, 443-469-8274 (Walk 23)

William Watson Statue W. North Ave. and W. Mount Royal Ave. (Walk 20)

William Welch Statue Johns Hopkins University, Shriver Hall (Walk 25)

MUSEUMS

American Visionary Art Museum avam.org, 800 Key Hwy., 410-244-1900 (Walk 3)

The Babe Ruth Birthplace and Museum baberuthmuseum.com, 216 Emory St., 410-727-1539 (Walk 13)

The Baltimore Museum of Art artbma.org, 10 Art Museum Dr., 443-573-1700 (Walk 25)

Baltimore Streetcar Museum baltimorestreetcar.org, 1901 Falls Rd., 410-547-0264 (Walk 22)

Baltimore Tattoo Museum baltimoretattoomuseum.net, 1534 Eastern Ave., 410-522-5800 (Walk 6)

B&O Railroad Museum borail.org, 901 W. Pratt St., 410-752-2490 (Walk 14)

Carroll Mansion carrollmuseums.org, 800 E. Lombard St., 410-605-2964 (Walk 10)

The Contemporary Museum contemporary.org (Walk 16)

The Dr. Samuel D. Harris National Museum of Dentistry dentalmuseum.org, 31 S. Greene St., 410-706-0600 (Walk 13)

Edgar Allan Poe House 203 N. Amity St., 410-396-4883 (Walk 14)

Evergreen Museum & Library museums.jhu.edu/evergreen.php, 4545 N. Charles St., 410-516-0341 (Walk 29)

Frederick Douglass–Isaac Myers Maritime Park douglassmyers.org, 1417 Thames St., 410-685-0295 (Walk 6)

Geppi's Entertainment Museum geppismuseum.com, 301 W. Camden St., 410-625-7060 (Walk 11, Walk 13)

H. L. Mencken House (Friends of the H. L. Mencken House) menckenhouse.org, 1524 Hollins St. (Walk 14)

Homewood House Museum museums.jhu.edu/homewood, Johns Hopkins University, 3400 N. Charles St., 410-516-5589 (Walk 25)

Irish Shrine Museum irishshrine.org, 918 and 920 Lemmon St., 410-669-8154 (Walk 14)

The Jewish Museum of Maryland jhsm.org, 15 Lloyd St., 410-732-6400 (Walk 10)

The Lacrosse Museum & National Hall of Fame uslacrosse.org/museum/halloffame, 113 W. University Pkwy, 410-235-6882 (Walk 25)

Mount Clare Museum House mountclare.org, Carroll Park, 1500 Washington Blvd., 410-837-3262 (Walk 15)

Museum of Industry thebmi.org, 1415 Key Hwy., 410-727-4808 (Walk 4)

National Pinball Museum nationalpinballmuseum.org, 608 Water St., 443-438-1241 (Walk 5)

Port Discovery Children's Museum portdiscovery.org, 35 Market Pl., 410-727-8120 (Walk 5)

President Street Station/Baltimore Civil War Museum 601 President St., 443-220-0290 (Walk 5)

The Reginald F. Lewis Museum of Maryland African American History & Culture 830 E. Pratt St., 443-263-1800 (Walk 5)

Sports Legends Museum baberuthmuseum.com/history/slmacy, 301 W. Camden St., 410-727-1539 (Walk 11, Walk 13)

The Walters Art Museum thewalters.org, 600 N. Charles St., 410-547-9000 (Walk 16)

Outdoor recreation & Parks

Canton Waterfront Park 2903 Boston St. (Walk 7)

Druid Hill Park/Jones Falls Trail Friends of Druid Hill Park, druidhillpark.org, 443-469-8274 (Walk 23, Walk 28)

Federal Hill Park Battery and Warren Aves. (Walk 3)

Gwynns Falls Trail gwynnsfallstrail.org, 410-448-5663, ext. 135 (Walk 2, Walk 15)

Herring Run Park 3800 Bel Air Rd. (Walk 26)

Lake Montebello Lake Dr. (Walk 26)

Mt. Washington Arboretum miniarboretum.org, Village of Mt. Washington (Walk 32)

Patterson Park pattersonpark.com, 27 S. Patterson Park Ave., 410-276-3676 (Walk 9)

Sherwood Gardens guilfordassociation.org/sherwood; Greenway, Stratford Rd., Highfield Rd., and Underwood Rd. (Walk 29)

Public art, arts institutions, & architecture

Alex Brown Building 135 E. Baltimore St. (Walk 12)

Baltimore City Hall baltimorecity.gov, 100 N. Holliday St. (Walk 12)

Baltimore Street Bridge W. Baltimore St. (between 2500 and 2900 blocks) (Walk 15)

Bank of America Building 10 Light St. (Walk 12)

Bromo Seltzer Arts Tower bromoseltzertower.com, 21 S. Eutaw St., 443-874-3596 (Walk 13)

Carrollton Viaduct Gwynns Falls near Carroll Park (Walk 15)

Cedarcroft School cedarcroftschool.com, 419 Cedarcroft Rd., 410-435-0905 (Walk 33)

Creative Alliance creativealliance.org, 3134 Eastern Ave., 410-276-1651 (Walk 9)

Customs House 40 S. Gay St. (Walk 12)

Eastern Avenue Underpass Between S. Haven St. and S. Lehigh St. (Walk 8)

Equitable Building 10 N. Calvert St. (Walk 12)

Fifth Regiment Armory 219 29th Division St., 410-576-6097 (Walk 20)

Garrett-Jacobs Mansion/Engineers Club garrettjacobsmansion.org, 11 W. Mount Vernon Pl.,
410-539-6914 (Walk 16)

Hansa Haus E. Redwood and Charles Sts. (Walk 12)

The McKim School 1120 E. Baltimore St. (Walk 10)

Mercantile Deposit & Trust Co. Building 200 E. Redwood St. (Walk 12)

Montgomery Park 1800 Washington Blvd. (Walk 15)

Moorish Tower Druid Hill Park (Walk 23)

Munsey Building 7 N. Calvert St. (Walk 12)

Octagon House acc-mtwashingtonconferencecenter.com, Mt. Washington Conference Center,
5801 Smith Ave., 800-488-8734 (Walk 32)

Old Town Friends' Meeting House 1201 E. Fayette St. (Walk 10)

Patterson Park Pagoda (The Friends of Patterson Park) pattersonpark.com,
27 S. Patterson Park Ave., 410-276-3676 (Walk 9)

Peabody Institute of The Johns Hopkins University peabody.jhu.edu, 1 E. Mount Vernon Pl.,
410-234-4500 (Walk 16)

Peabody Library peabodyevents.library.jhu.edu, 17 E. Mount Vernon Pl., 410-234-4943 (Walk 16)

Penn Station 1500 N. Charles St. (Walk 21)

Phoenix Shot Tower 801 E. Fayette St., 410-837-5424 (Walk 10)

Roland Park Fire House Upland Rd. (Walk 30)

Rolando-Thom Mansion 204 W. Lanvale St. (Walk 19)

Romare Bearden Mural Upton Metro Station, Pennsylvania Ave. (Walk 17)

Stone Hill Historic District Pacific, Puritan, Bay, Field, and Worth Sts. (Walk 27)

University of Maryland School of Medicine Davidge Hall medschool.umaryland.edu/davidge, 522 W. Lombard St. (Walk 13)

Washington Monument and Museum at Mount Vernon Place 699 N. Charles St., 410-396-1049 (Walk 16)

Westminster Hall westminsterhall.org, 519 W. Fayette St., 410-706-2072 (Walk 13)

SHOPPING/DINING/COMMERCIAL DEVELOPMENTS

American Can Company thecancompany.com, 2400 Boston St., 443-573-4460 (Walk 7)

Belvedere Square belvederesquare.com, 518 E. Belvedere Ave., 410-464-9773 (Walk 33)

Brewers Hill brewershill.net, Conkling Street to O'Donnell and Dillon Sts. (Walk 7)

Clipper Mill clippermillbaltimore.com, Clipper Mill Road (Walk 28)

Meadow Mill Clipper Mill Road (Walk 28)

Mt. Washington Mill mtwashingtonmill.com, 1340 Smith Ave., 410-385-1234 (Walk 32)

O'Donnell Square 2900 block of O'Donnell St. (Walk 7)

Tudor Shopping Center Upland Rd. and Roland Ave. (Walk 30)

Union Mill theunionmill.com, 1500 Union Ave., 443-682-9945 (Walk 28)

INDEX

aBOUT THE aUTHOr

Evan L. Balkan teaches writing at the Community College of Baltimore County. He is the author of five previous books of nonfiction, including *60 Hikes Within 60 Miles: Baltimore* and *Best Tent Camping: Maryland*. His latest book is *The Wrath of God: Lope de Aguirre, Revolutionary of the Americas*. He holds degrees from Towson, George Mason, and Johns Hopkins Universities and lives in Towson, Maryland, with his wife and two daughters.

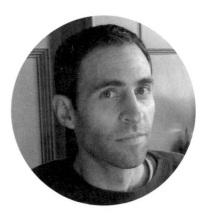